50 Studies Every Occupational Therapist Should Know

50 STUDIES EVERY DOCTOR SHOULD KNOW

50 Studies Every Doctor Should Know: The Key Studies that Form the Foundation of Evidence Based Medicine, Revised Edition
Michael E. Hochman

50 Studies Every Internist Should Know
Kristopher Swiger, Joshua R. Thomas, Michael E. Hochman, and Steven Hochman

50 Studies Every Neurologist Should Know
David Y. Hwang and David M. Greer

50 Studies Every Pediatrician Should Know
Ashaunta T. Anderson, Nina L. Shapiro, Stephen C. Aronoff, Jeremiah Davis, and Michael Levy

50 Imaging Studies Every Doctor Should Know
Christoph I. Lee

50 Studies Every Surgeon Should Know
SreyRam Kuy, Rachel J. Kwon, and Miguel A. Burch

50 Studies Every Intensivist Should Know
Edward A. Bittner

50 Studies Every Palliative Care Doctor Should Know
David Hui, Akhila Reddy, and Eduardo Bruera

50 Studies Every Psychiatrist Should Know
Ish P. Bhalla, Rajesh R. Tampi, and Vinod H. Srihari

50 Studies Every Anesthesiologist Should Know
Anita Gupta, Michael E. Hochman, and Elena N. Gutman

50 Studies Every Ophthalmologist Should Know
Alan D. Penman, Kimberly W. Crowder, and William M. Watkins, Jr.

50 Studies Every Urologist Should Know
Philipp Dahm

50 Studies Every Obstetrician and Gynecologist Should Know
Constance Liu, Noah Rindos, and Scott Shainker

50 Studies Every Doctor Should Know: The Key Studies that Form the Foundation of Evidence-Based Medicine, 2nd Edition
Michael E. Hochman and Steven D. Hochman

50 Studies Every Occupational Therapist Should Know
Elizabeth A. Pyatak and Elissa S. Lee

50 Studies Every Occupational Therapist Should Know

EDITED BY

ELIZABETH A. PYATAK, PHD, OTR/L, CDCES, FAOTA
Associate Professor
Chan Division of Occupational Science and Occupational Therapy
University of Southern California
Los Angeles, CA, USA

ELISSA S. LEE, OTD, OTR
Clinical Strategy Manager
SCAN Health Plan
Long Beach, CA, USA

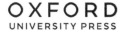

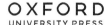

Oxford University Press is a department of the University of Oxford. It furthers
the University's objective of excellence in research, scholarship, and education
by publishing worldwide. Oxford is a registered trade mark of Oxford University
Press in the UK and certain other countries.

Published in the United States of America by Oxford University Press
198 Madison Avenue, New York, NY 10016, United States of America.

Library of Congress Cataloging-in-Publication Data
Names: Pyatak, Elizabeth A, editor. | Lee, Elissa S., editor.
Title: 50 studies every occupational therapist should know / [edited by] Elizabeth Pyatak A, Elissa S. Lee.
Other titles: Fifty studies every occupational therapist should know |
50 studies every doctor should know (Series)
Description: New York, NY : Oxford University Press, [2023] |
Series: 50 studies every doctor should know |
Includes bibliographical references and index.
Identifiers: LCCN 2022027474 (print) | LCCN 2022027475 (ebook) |
ISBN 9780197630402 (paperback) | ISBN 9780197630426 (epub) | ISBN 9780197630433 (online)
Subjects: MESH: Occupational Therapy—methods |
Evidence-Based Medicine—methods | Case Reports
Classification: LCC RM735.3 (print) | LCC RM735.3 (ebook) | NLM WB 555 |
DDC 615.8/515—dc23/eng/20220817
LC record available at https://lccn.loc.gov/2022027474
LC ebook record available at https://lccn.loc.gov/2022027475

DOI: 10.1093/med/9780197630402.001.0001

9 8 7 6 5 4 3 2 1

Printed by Marquis, Canada

CONTENTS

SECTION 6 Rehabilitation and Disability

CONTRIBUTORS

Yasaman Amanat, OTD, OTR/L, CLT
Assistant Professor of Clinical
  Occupational Therapy
Chan Division of Occupational
  Science and Occupational Therapy
University of Southern California
Los Angeles, CA, USA

Arameh Anvarizadeh, OTD, OTR/L, FAOTA
Director of Admissions/Associate
  Professor of Clinical Occupational
  Therapy
Chan Division of Occupational
  Science and Occupational Therapy
University of Southern California
Los Angeles, CA, USA

Sajay Arthanat, PhD, OTR/L, ATP
Professor
Department of Occupational Therapy
The University of New Hampshire
Durham, NH, USA

Karla K. Ausderau, PhD, OTR/L
Associate Professor/Waisman Center
  Investigator
Department of Kinesiology,
  Occupational Therapy Program
Waisman Center
University of Wisconsin–Madison
Madison, WI, USA

Soyoung Esther Bae, OTD, OTR/L
Occupational Therapist
Los Angeles County Department of
  Mental Health
Los Angeles, CA, USA

Teal W. Benevides, PhD, MS, OTR/L
Associate Professor, Institute of Public
  and Preventive Health
Augusta University
Augusta, GA, USA

Erna I. Blanche, PhD, OTR/L, FAOTA
Clinical Professor of Occupational
  Therapy
Chan Division of Occupational
  Science and Occupational Therapy
University of Southern California
Los Angeles, CA, USA

Stefanie Bodison, OTD, OTR/L
Assistant Professor
Department of Occupational Therapy
College of Public Health and Health
  Professions
University of Florida
Gainesville, FL, USA

Kristine Carandang, PhD, OTR/L
Research Scientist
Young Patients' Autoimmune
  Research & Empowerment Alliance
River Falls, WI, USA

**Sharon A. Cermak, EdD, OTR/L,
FAOTA**
Professor of Occupational Science
  and Occupational Therapy
Chan Division of Occupational
  Science and Occupational Therapy
Professor of Pediatrics
Keck School of Medicine
University of Southern California
Los Angeles, CA, USA

**Megan C. Chang, PhD, OTR/L,
FAOTA**
Associate Professor
San José State University
San José, CA, USA

Candace Chatman, OTD, OTR/L
Assistant Professor of Clinical
  Occupational Therapy
Chan Division of Occupational
  Science and Occupational Therapy
University of Southern California
Los Angeles, CA, USA

Allison Chu, OTD, OTR/L
Associate Professor of Clinical
  Occupational Therapy
Chan Division of Occupational
  Science and Occupational Therapy
University of Southern California
Los Angeles, CA, USA

**Dominique H. Como, PhD,
EdM, OTR/L**
Research Assistant
Chan Division of Occupational
  Science and Occupational Therapy
University of Southern California
Los Angeles, CA, USA

**Rebecca Cunningham, OTD,
OTR/L, MSCS**
Chan Division of Occupational
  Science and Occupational Therapy
University of Southern California
Los Angeles, CA, USA

**Jessica De Brun, OTD, MOT,
OTR/L**
Assistant Professor
University of St. Augustine for Health
  Sciences
San Marcos, CA, USA

Jesus Diaz, OTD, OTR/L
Associate Chair of Diversity, Access,
  and Equity
Associate Professor of Research
Chan Division of Occupational
  Science and Occupational Therapy
University of Southern California
Los Angeles, CA, USA

Beth Fields, PhD, OTR/L, BCG
Assistant Professor
Department of Kinesiology
University of Wisconsin—Madison
Madison, WI, USA

Marshae D. Franklin, OTD, OTR/L
PhD Student
Chan Division of Occupational
    Science and Occupational Therapy
University of Southern California
Los Angeles, CA, USA

Heather Fritz, PhD, OTR/L, CHC
Assistant Professor and Founding
    Director
School of Occupational Therapy
Pacific Northwest University of
    Health Sciences
Yakima, WA, USA

Yoko E. Fukumura, MA, OTR/L
PhD Student/Research Assistant
Chan Division of Occupational
    Science and Occupational Therapy
University of Southern California
Los Angeles, CA, USA

**Tara J. Glennon, EdD, OTR/L,
FAOTA**
Professor
Department of Occupational Therapy
Quinnipiac University
Hamden, CT, USA

Cristin Holland, PhD, OTR/L
Postdoctoral Research Fellow
Department of Psychiatry
Columbia University Irving
    Medical Center
New York, NY, USA

Yi-Ling Hu, PhD, OTR/L
Assistant Professor
Department of Occupational Therapy
Chang Gung University
Taoyuan, Taiwan

Lisa Jaegers, PhD, OTR/L, FAOTA
Associate Professor
Department of Occupational Science
    and Occupational Therapy
Doisy College of Health Sciences
School of Social Work & Criminology
College for Public Health and Social
    Justice
Saint Louis University
St. Louis, MO, USA

**Katie Jordan, OTD, OTR/L,
FAOTA**
Associate Chair of Clinical
    Occupational Therapy Services
Professor of Clinical Occupational
    Therapy
Chan Division of Occupational
    Science and Occupational Therapy
University of Southern California
Los Angeles, CA, USA

Carlos Juarez Aguilar, OTR/L
Occupational Therapist
Project 180 LA
Los Angeles, CA, USA

Karrie Kingsley, OTD, OTR/L
Associate Professor of Clinical
    Occupational Therapy
Chan Division of Occupational
    Science and Occupational Therapy
University of Southern California
Los Angeles, CA, USA

**Carol Lambdin-Pattavina, OTD,
MSOT, OTR/L, CTP**
Assistant Professor
University of New England
Portland, ME, USA

Alison E. Lane, PhD, OTR
Professor
Olga Tennison Autism Research Centre
La Trobe University
Melbourne, Victoria, Australia

Elissa S. Lee, OTD, OTR
Clinical Strategy Manager
SCAN Health Plan
Long Beach, CA, USA

Chiung-ju Liu, PhD, OTR/L, FGSA
Associate Professor
Department of Occupational Therapy
University of Florida
Gainesville, FL, USA

Jenny Martínez, OTD, OTR/L, BCG, FAOTA
Associate Professor
Department of Occupational Therapy
Thomas Jefferson University
Philadelphia, PA, USA

Erin McIntyre, OTD, MA, OTR/L
Assistant Professor
University of St. Augustine for Health
  Sciences
San Marcos, CA, USA

Julie McLaughlin Gray, PhD, OTR/L, FAOTA
Associate Chair for Curriculum and
  Faculty
Professor of Clinical Occupational
  Therapy
Chan Division of Occupational
  Science and Occupational Therapy
University of Southern California
Los Angeles, CA, USA

Tessa Z. Milman, OTD, OTR/L
Assistant Professor of Clinical
  Occupational Therapy
Chan Division of Occupational
  Science and Occupational Therapy
University of Southern California
Los Angeles, CA, USA

Stacey Morikawa, OTD, OTR/L
Associate Professor of Clinical
  Occupational Therapy
Chan Division of Occupational
  Science and Occupational Therapy
University of Southern California
Los Angeles, CA, USA

Rashelle Nagata, OTD, OTR/L
Learning Specialist
Kaiser Permanente Bernard J. Tyson
  School of Medicine
Pasadena, CA, USA

Phuong Nguyen, OTD, OTR/L, CLT, Neuro-IFRAH® Certified Instructor
Associate Professor of Clinical
  Occupational Therapy
Chan Division of Occupational
  Science and Occupational Therapy
University of Southern California
Assistant Director of Occupational
  Therapy
Keck Medicine of USC
Los Angeles, CA, USA

Daniel Padilla Vega, OTD, OTR/L
Project 180
Los Angeles, CA, USA

Karen Park, OTD, OTR/L, BCP, SWC
Assistant Professor/Doctoral
  Coordinator
University of St. Augustine for Health
  Sciences
San Marcos, CA, USA

Andrew C. Persch, PhD, OTR/L, BCP
Associate Professor
Department of Occupational Therapy
Colorado State University
Fort Collins, CO, USA

Kelsey Peterson, OTD, OTR/L, Neuro-IFRAH° Certified Instructor
Assistant Professor of Clinical
  Occupational Therapy
Chan Division of Occupational
  Science and Occupational Therapy
University of Southern California
Los Angeles, CA, USA

Beth Pfeiffer, PhD, OTR/L, BCP, FAOTA
Associate Professor
Department of Health and
  Rehabilitation Sciences
Temple University
Philadelphia, PA, USA

Kaelah Pou, OTD, OTR/L
Occupational Therapist
District of Columbia Public Schools
Washington, DC, USA

Elizabeth A. Pyatak, PhD, OTR/L, CDCES, FAOTA
Associate Professor
Chan Division of Occupational
  Science and Occupational Therapy
University of Southern California
Los Angeles, CA, USA

Samia H. Rafeedie, OTD, OTR/L, BCPR, CBIS
Director of the Occupational Therapy
  Professional Program
Associate Professor of Clinical
  Occupational Therapy
Chan Division of Occupational
  Science and Occupational Therapy
University of Southern California
Los Angeles, CA, USA

Gustavo Reinoso, Ph.D., OTR/L
Associate Professor
Nova Southeastern University
Department of Occupational Therapy
Dr. Pallavi Patel College of Health
  Care Sciences
Clearwater, FL, USA

Stacey Reynolds PhD, OTR/L, FAOTA
Professor
Department of Occupational Therapy
Virginia Commonwealth University
Richmond, VA, USA

Pamela Roberts, PhD, OTR/L, SCFES, FAOTA, CPHQ, FNAP, FACRM
Executive Director and Professor
Physical Medicine and Rehabilitation
  and Medical Affairs
Cedars-Sinai
Los Angeles, CA, USA

Shawn C. Roll, PhD, OTR/L, RMSKS, FAOTA, FAIUM
Associate Professor
Chan Division of Occupational
  Science and Occupational Therapy
University of Southern California
Los Angeles, CA, USA

Preethy S. Samuel, PhD, OTR/L
Associate Professor
Department of Health Care Sciences
Wayne State University
Detroit, MI, USA

**Stacey L. Schepens Niemiec, PhD,
OTR/L, DipACLM/DipIBLM**
Associate Professor of Research
Chan Division of Occupational
   Science and Occupational Therapy
University of Southern California
Los Angeles, CA, USA

**Arlene A. Schmid, PhD,
OTR, FAOTA**
Professor
Department of Occupational Therapy
Colorado State University
Fort Collins, CO, USA

Tristan Scremin, JD, MFA
Community Liaison
Painted Brain
Expert by Experience
Chan Division of Occupational
   Science and Occupational Therapy
University of Southern California
Los Angeles, CA, USA

Carol Siebert, OTD, OT/L, FAOTA
Founder/CEO
The Home Remedy PLLC/
   Occupational Therapy
Chapel Hill, NC, USA

**Alix G. Sleight, PhD, OTD,
MPH, OTR/L**
Clinical Scientist
Department of Physical Medicine and
   Rehabilitation
Center for Integrated Research in
   Cancer and Lifestyle
Samuel Oschin Cancer Center
Cedars-Sinai
Los Angeles, CA, USA

**Jeff Snodgrass, PhD, MPH,
OTR, FAOTA**
Associate Dean of Academic Affairs,
   Professor
College of Clinical and Rehabilitative
   Health Sciences
East Tennessee State University
Johnson City, TN, USA

Leah I. Stein Duker, PhD, OTR/L
Assistant Professor of Research
Chan Division of Occupational
   Science and Occupational Therapy
University of Southern California
Los Angeles, CA, USA

Kayoko Takahashi, ScD, OTR
Professor, School of Allied Health
   Sciences
Kitasato University
Kanagawa, Japan

**Ana Verran, MA, OTR/L,
SCDCM, CDRS**
Research Adjunct Professor (Ret.)
Chan Division of Occupational
   Science and Occupational Therapy
University of Southern California
Los Angeles, CA, USA

Rafael Wagas, OTD, OTRP, OTR/L, CDP
Occupational Therapy Supervisor
Powerback Rehabilitation
Sacramento, CA, USA

Selena Washington, PhD, MSPH, OTR/L
Department of Occupational Science
   and Occupational Therapy
Doisy College of Health Sciences
Saint Louis University
St. Louis, MO, USA

Renee Watling, PhD, OTR/L, FAOTA
Clinical Assistant Professor
University of Puget Sound
Tacoma, WA, USA

INTRODUCTION

A common rite of passage among occupational therapy (OT) students and practitioners[1] is developing an "elevator speech" of what constitutes our profession, which is often unfamiliar to our colleagues, clients, and closest loved ones. This book illustrates why the question "What is OT?" is so challenging to answer as we attempt to capture the range of OT literature with 50 studies that reveal the myriad dimensions of our practice.

To tackle the complexity of OT practice, we used six key practice areas as outlined by the American Occupational Therapy Association as a heuristic for classifying studies to include in the book: (1) productive aging, (2) health and wellness, (3) work and industry, (4) mental health, (5) children and youth, and (6) rehabilitation and disability. These sections were edited by experts in the field, who in turn invited authors with varied perspectives and expertise to contribute individual chapters. Furthermore, section editors provided introductions to contextualize their study choices and areas of practice (a first for the 50 Studies series!).

As we identified studies for this book, we were guided by demonstrable indicators of significance and impact, such as citation rate, rigor of the research design, or having influenced OT practice, policy, or legislation. We also sought to represent the breadth of OT practice, rather than focusing more narrowly on what might be considered the most rigorous or trustworthy studies within our profession. In making this decision, we accepted that this would lead to significant variability, both within and across practice areas, in terms of the nature and type of research available on a given subject. Rather than seeking out methodologically perfect studies irrespective of their impact on the field, we endeavored

---

1 This text uses both "occupational therapist" and "occupational therapy practitioner" to refer to individuals who are licensed and qualified to provide occupational therapy services.

to paint a landscape of where OT literature and practice stand today. After the editors and section editors chose studies to be considered for inclusion, the list of candidate studies underwent anonymous expert peer review to ensure their relevance and importance to the field, which informed the final 50 studies.

While our anthology of studies does not necessarily reflect the commonly understood "gold standard" for evidence in healthcare, we also challenge this paradigm as the foundation for high-quality care. To improve the lives of those we serve, we advocate both for rigorous research providing empirical evidence of OT's efficacy and for trustworthy qualitative research that offers perspective on how lived experience influences health and well-being.

We encouraged authors and section editors throughout the process to critically examine and incorporate a diversity of perspectives that would be culturally and clinically relevant to historically marginalized individuals and communities. While reading this book, we would invite you to reflect on the state of the evidence informing healthcare delivery today and the degree to which it is equitable and provides a foundation for OT practice within our diverse society.

Toward that end, we consider this book as a work in progress and envision? that when the book has future editions, the realm of available studies will continue to evolve and expand. We anticipate seeing more research casting a critical lens on OT practice, in particular our continued emphasis on independence, productivity, and individualism as influenced by Western values; more studies conducted by, and with, communities that have been historically excluded from knowledge creation that is institutionally recognized and funded; and more high-level evidence that will be persuasive to payors, policy makers, and other stakeholders of the value of our profession. In advocating for these changes, we join Hammell (2009) in her healthy skepticism regarding the universality of our assumptions around occupation and Lavelley and Johnson (2020) in recognizing occupation as a tool for reinforcing occupational injustice and justice across the United States and in the world.

The process of developing this book has provided us with a renewed appreciation of the intricacies and nuances of OT practice, both historically and in the present day, and has shaped our vision for the future. As the first 50 Studies book to represent a health profession outside of medicine, we are proud to provide an overview for both OT students and practitioners as well as others interested in better understanding our profession.

While there may never be a definitive answer to the question "What is OT?" we hope this book provides you a new perspective on OT practice, its impact on the people we serve, and its evolving place in the greater healthcare field.

References

Hammell, K. W. (2009). Sacred texts: A sceptical exploration of the assumptions underpinning theories of occupation. *Canadian Journal of Occupational Therapy, 76*(1), 6–13.

Lavalley, R., & Johnson, K. R. (2020). Occupation, injustice, and anti-Black racism in the United States of America. *Journal of Occupational Science*. Advance online publication. https://doi.org/10.1080/14427591.2020.1810111

SECTION 1

Productive Aging

By the year 2050, one in every six people in the world is expected to be an older adult (65 years or older) (United Nations Department of Economic and Social Affairs, 2019). Alongside the opportunities afforded by increased longevity and decline in mortality is the challenge of rising multimorbidity across the globe. More than 66% of older adults live with more than one chronic condition (Ofori-Asenso et al., 2019), which increases the likelihood of developing functional limitations and disability that often significantly detract from quality of life. This has drawn necessary attention to how society can successfully adapt to population aging and capitalize on opportunities to build a vibrant older population. Discussions about life span have steadily transitioned to "healthspan"—the years of life during which one enjoys health and well-being, free from chronic disease and disability (Kaeberlein, 2018). From an occupational lens, productive aging "celebrate[s] older adults' capabilities, potential, and social and economic contributions" (Misey Boyer, 2007, p. 8). Occupational therapy (OT) brings distinct value to productive aging by facilitating participation in meaningful occupations, promoting health and well-being, and offering cost-effective, client-centered solutions that result in positive health outcomes (American Occupational Therapy Association, 2016).

This section of the book curates some of the most important research regarding OT interventions that foster productive aging. A broad search for intervention studies relevant to productive aging was undertaken; following expert peer review, nine articles were selected for final inclusion. Although not representative of every topic originally searched, primary domains ultimately covered in this section are falls and falls prevention, home modifications, health promotion and wellness, and chronic disease management. Additional areas addressed to some degree within these articles include activities of daily living (ADLs), instrumental ADLs, and technology. Studies took place in Western contexts (i.e., the United States, the Netherlands, Australia, the United Kingdom). Ethnoracial makeup of the samples was only reported in the US studies; all others were presumably composed of non-Latino/Hispanic White older adults. Generally, study populations included predominantly White participants (Gitlin et al., Mann et al., Tennstedt et al.), with the exception of Clark et al. (64% of participants were non-White—mostly Asian) and Szanton et al. (79% were Black), highlighting the need to continue efforts to increase diversity within research studies.

As evident in this section, OT has excelled in the interconnected areas of falls prevention and home safety/modification. Clemson et al.'s, Tennstedt et al.'s, and Close et al.'s studies tackled the complexity of falls—each demonstrating significant psychosocial and health benefits—with divergent approaches to intervention. Relevant to falls prevention, Mann et al.'s and Szanton et al.'s works focused on home safety and function. Aligned with the falls prevention and home modification research that contributed to aging in place, Clark et al.'s groundbreaking Well Elderly Study introduced to the profession preventative OT for community-living older adults. Graff et al.'s and Gitlin et al.'s studies honed in on a narrower population—older adults with dementia and their care partners—incorporating in-home skill-building and activity participation. Sturkenboom et al.'s work also featured a home-based program but for persons with Parkinson's disease and involved strategy-building and task and environmental adaptations.

The studies in this section have created a strong foundation for current and future intervention research in productive aging. These impactful studies support the efficacy of OT to facilitate productive aging and strengthen OT's role in this ever-growing and increasingly important domain.

References

American Occupational Therapy Association. (2016). *Occupational therapy's distinct value: Productive aging.* Retrieved May 28, 2021, from https://www.aota.org/-/media/Corporate/Files/Practice/Aging/Distinct-Value-Productive-Aging.pdf

Kaeberlein, M. (2018). How healthy is the healthspan concept? *Geroscience, 40*(4), 361–364.

Misey Boyer, J. (2007). *Creativity matters: The arts and aging toolkit*. National Guild of Community Schools of the Arts.

Ofori-Asenso, R., Chin, K. L., Curtis, A. J., Zomer, E., Zoungas, S., & Liew, D. (2019). Recent patterns of multimorbidity among older adults in high-income countries. *Population Health Management, 22*(2), 127–137.

United Nations Department of Economic and Social Affairs. (2019). *World population prospects 2019*. Retrieved May 28, 2021, from https://population.un.org/wpp/

1

Preventing Falls by Integrating Functional Exercise into Habitual Daily Routines

YI-LING HU AND CHIUNG-JU LIU

The LiFE study

LiFE is a tailored programme of embedded balance and strength activities, taught over five home visits with two booster visits. It was designed to reduce fall risk and resulted in a clinically important 31% reduction in the rate of falls compared with the control programme.

CLEMSON, L., SINGH, M. A. F., BUNDY, A., CUMMING, R. G., MANOLLARAS, K., O'LOUGHLIN, P., & BLACK, D. (2012). Integration of balance and strength training into daily life activity to reduce rate of falls in older people (the LiFE study): Randomised parallel trial. BMJ, 345, Article e4547.

Original Paper: https://www.bmj.com/content/345/bmj.E4547

The LiFE Program Trainers' and Participants' Manuals: https://www.sydney.edu.au/medicine-health/schools/sydney-school-of-health-sciences/academic-staff/lindy-clemson.html

Research Question: Is the Lifestyle-integrated Functional Exercise (LiFE) program more effective in preventing falls among high-risk older adults living at home compared to structured strength and balance exercise and gentle flexibility exercise?

Funding: The National Health and Medical Research Council in Australia.

Year Study Began: 2006

Year Study Published: 2012

Study Location: Metropolitan Sydney, Australia

Who Was Studied: Older adults (aged 70 years or above) at risk for falls (self-reported two or more falls or one injurious fall in the past 12 months).

Who Was Excluded: Older adults who had moderate to severe cognitive problems, were unable to ambulate independently, had neurological conditions that severely influenced gait and mobility, resided in a nursing home or hostel, or had an unstable or terminal illness that would preclude exercise.

How Many Patients: 317

Study Overview: See Figure 1.1.

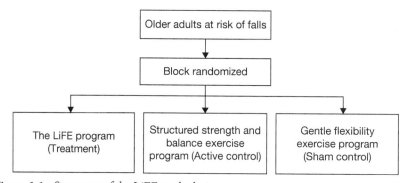

Figure 1.1. Summary of the LiFE study design.

Study Intervention: The LiFE program embeds exercise in everyday activities, rather than as a structured program. Older adults in the treatment group performed the LiFE program whenever the opportunity arose during the day. Participants learned strategies from the LiFE program to challenge balance (e.g., reduce base of support, shift weight from foot to foot) and increase leg strength (e.g., bend your knees, raise up on your toes) and incorporated these strategies in everyday activities. An example of an integrated leg strengthening activity is squatting instead of bending at the waist to close a drawer.

Older adults in the active control group performed structured exercise activities, which included seven balance exercises and six lower limb strength exercises three times a week.

Older adults in the sham control group performed 12 gentle and flexibility exercises.

Follow-Up: 12 months

Endpoints: Primary endpoint: Number of falls over 12 months as measured by self-report. Secondary endpoints:

- Static balance as measured using two hierarchical balance scales
- Dynamic balance as measured by 3-m tandem walk test
- Ankle muscle strength as measured using as dynamometer
- Balance confidence as measured by Activities-Specific Balance Confidence Scale
- Activities of daily living as measured by National Health and Nutrition Examination Survey (NHANES) independence measure for activities of daily life
- Adherence rate as measured by weekly self-report logs

RESULTS

- The overall incidence of falls in the LiFE program was 1.66 per person-years, compared with 1.90 in the structured balance and strength exercise program and 2.28 in the gentle flexibility exercise program.
- Older adults in the LiFE program:
  - Showed a clinically important reduction of 31% in the rate of falls compared with those in the gentle flexibility exercise program.
  - Significantly improved in static balance and ankle strength compared with those in the other two programs (Table 1.1).
  - Significantly improved in activities of daily living based on the NHANES measure compared with those in the gentle flexibility exercise program (Table 1.1).
- Older adults in the LiFE program as well as the structured balance and strength exercise program showed significant gains in balance confidence compared to those in the gentle flexibility exercise program (Table 1.1).

- The adherence rate in the LiFE program was higher at 12 months (64%) compared with the structured balance and strength exercise (53%) and the gentle flexibility exercise programs (53%).

Table 1.1. LiFE Program Outcomes

	LiFE versus Gentle Exercise Effect Size (p)	Structured Exercise versus Gentle Exercise Effect Size (p)
Static balance (eight-level hierarchy)	0.63 (<0.001)*	0.29 (0.08)
Ankle strength (right)	0.40 (0.005)*	0.26 (0.10)
Ankle strength (left)	0.40 (<0.0001)*	0.17 (0.34)
Balance confidence	0.38 (0.004)*	0.37 (0.006)*
Activities of daily living	0.54 (<0.0001)*	0.26 (0.075)

Criticisms and Limitations: It is unclear whether physical activity not prescribed as a part of the LiFE program was tracked or analyzed. For example, participants in the LiFE program might have begun engaging in structured physical exercises during the intervention period in addition to LiFE program activities, which would confound outcomes.

Other Relevant Studies and Information:

- A pragmatic randomized controlled trial in older adults receiving restorative home care services in Australia has rendered similar results. Participants in the LiFE group improved in more balance and functional outcomes than those in a structured exercise group after the intervention (95% vs. 70%) (Burton et al., 2013). Additionally, participants in the LiFE group continued to show progress in 25% of the outcomes 6 months after the intervention had ended (Burton et al., 2014).
- Behavior change techniques have been incorporated into the LiFE program and tested in middle-aged and older women. The results showed that the techniques increased action and automaticity (Fleig et al., 2016).
- The LiFE program has been tested in people with vision impairment and demonstrated good feasibility and acceptability (Keay et al., 2015).
- The LiFE program has been adapted for a more diverse population in the United States. A mixed method study showed preliminary feasibility with high acceptance to adapt LiFE for Black older adults (Hu et al., 2020).

Summary and Implications: The LiFE program principles are to increase the physical demands of daily activity by challenging balance and lower extremity strength during everyday routines. The program yields high adherence and is effective in reducing falls in older adults, particularly those who are at high risk of falling. The LiFE program offers a novel alternative to structured exercise programs for fall prevention in late life.

CLINICAL CASE: LIFE PROGRAM FOR AN OLDER ADULT AT RISK OF FALLS

Case History

Delores (she/her), 72 years old, lives alone in a senior apartment. Delores retired as a bus driver 10 years ago, but she still takes care of her younger grandchildren on the weekends for her daughter. She enjoys family gatherings and going to church. Delores fell and broke her wrist when she missed a step as she descended stairs at her church last December. After the fall, she began limiting her activities outside of her home, fearing that if she was "too active," she might fall again. Unfortunately, Delores experienced a second fall last week in her apartment, only 9 months after her first fall. Although she neither suffered any injuries nor showed any signs of cognitive deficits this time, the results of her occupational therapy evaluations suggested fear of falling and reduced balance and muscle strength of the lower extremity. Is Delores a good candidate for the LiFE program? If yes, what would implementation of this program look like for Delores?

Suggested Answer

Delores would be a good candidate to receive the LiFE program. The program materials (a daily calendar and user manual) are recommended to teach Delores how to incorporate strategies that progressively challenge her balance and leg muscle strength into her daily routines. Delores can start by embedding one or two strategies into one of her routine daily activities. For example, she could practice narrow standing (a challenge to her balance) when she heats food in the microwave. Alternatively, Delores can engage in heel raises (a challenge to ankle muscle strength), using her fingertips for light support on the kitchen counter, while waiting for cookies to bake in the oven. The LiFE program will help restore Delores's balance confidence and prevent future falls by building a habit of integrating balance and leg strengthening activities whenever she sees an opportunity in her everyday routines.

References

Burton, E., Lewin, G., Clemson, L., & Boldy, D. (2013). Effectiveness of a lifestyle exercise program for older people receiving a restorative home care service: A pragmatic randomized controlled trial. *Clinical Interventions in Aging, 8*, 1591–1601. https://doi.org/10.2147/CIA.S44614

Burton, E., Lewin, G., Clemson, L., & Boldy, D. (2014). Long-term benefits of a lifestyle exercise program for older people receiving a restorative home care service: A pragmatic randomized controlled trial. *Healthy Aging & Clinical Care in the Elderly, 2014*(6), 1–9. https://doi.org/10.4137/HACCE.S13445

Fleig, L., McAllister, M. M., Chen, P., Iverson, J., Milne, K., McKay, H. A., Clemson, L., & Ashe, M. C. (2016). Health behaviour change theory meets falls prevention: Feasibility of a habit-based balance and strength exercise intervention for older adults. *Psychology of Sport and Exercise, 22*, 114–122. https://doi.org/10.1016/j.psychsport.2015.07.002

Hu, Y., Keglovits, M., Somerville, E., Snyder, M., & Stark, S. (2020). Translating a functional exercise program for fall prevention among diverse older adults in urban medically underserved areas: A mixed methods study. *Journal of Aging and Physical Activity, 29*(4), 612–619. https://journals.humankinetics.com/view/journals/japa/aop/article-10.1123-japa.2019-0159/article-10.1123-japa.2019-0159.xml

Keay, L., Saich, F., & Clemson, L. (2015). Feasibility and acceptability of orientation and mobility instructors delivering the LiFE falls prevention program to older people with vision impairment. *International Journal of Orientation & Mobility, 7*, 22–33. https://doi.org/10.21307/ijom-2017-053

2

Community-Based Group Intervention to Reduce Fear of Falling and Activity Restriction

ARLENE A. SCHMID

A Matter of Balance

The results of this study [...] have established the importance of fear of falling as a targeted outcome for intervention. The results of this trial indicate that short-term changes can be achieved in maladaptive attitudes and beliefs about falling and in activity levels and functioning.

> TENNSTEDT, S., HOWLAND, J., LACHMAN, M., PETERSON, E., KASTEN, L., & JETTE, A. (1998). A randomized, controlled trial of a group intervention to reduce fear of falling and associated activity restriction in older adults. *The Journals of Gerontology Series B: Psychological Sciences and Social Sciences*, 53(6), P384–P392.

Original Paper: https://academic.oup.com/psychsocgerontology/article/53B/6/P384/618638

Research Question: Does a group intervention (A Matter of Balance) decrease fear of falling while at the same time improving self-efficacy, a sense of control, and physical and social activity?

Funding: Boston University Roybal Center Consortium for Research in Applied Gerontology, funded by the National Institute on Aging

Year Study Began: 1994

Year Study Published: 1998

Study Location: Boston, MA

Who Was Studied: English-speaking adults aged 60 and over with a self-reported restriction in activity due to fear of falling who lived in senior housing.

- Average age was 78 years
- 9% were minorities
- Majority had less than high school education

Who Was Excluded: Older adults with a major physical or health condition that might have impeded engagement in the intervention.

How Many Patients: 434

Study Overview: Participants were randomized to A Matter of Balance intervention or the control group (social contact group) (Figure 2.1).

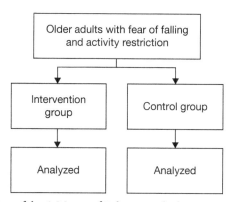

Figure 2.1. Overview of the A Matter of Balance study design.

Study Intervention: The A Matter of Balance intervention was delivered for 2 hours, twice a week for 4 weeks (eight sessions total). Using a cognitive restructuring approach, the standardized intervention was developed to promote activity by reducing fear of falling. The intervention addressed self-efficacy and attitudes and included videos, lectures, group discussion, problem-solving, role-playing, exercise, assertiveness training, home assignments, and behavioral contracting. The intervention was taught by two trained facilitators, and each group included approximately 11 participants.

The social contact control group met once for a 2-hour group session and was taught by the same trained facilitators as the intervention. The session included a presentation about falls incidence, fall risk factors, home hazards, and steps to reduce fall risk. Discussion took place but did not address fear of falling or activity restriction.

Follow-Up: Participants were tested at baseline, 6 weeks (after the 4-week intervention), and 6 and 12 months to assess sustainability.

Endpoints:

Primary outcomes:

- Falls self-efficacy was assessed with the modified version of the Falls Efficacy Scale.
- Perceived control over falling was assessed using a study-specific scale.
- Perceived ability to manage fall risk or falls was assessed with a study-specific scale.
- Number of falls was assessed by a single question about frequency of falls between sessions.

Secondary outcomes:

- Change in behavior due to health problems was assessed with the Sickness Impact Profile.
- Intended activity (plan to perform an activity in the next week) was assessed with the Intended Activity Scale.

Assessors were blinded to randomization.

RESULTS

- Overall, 434 participants were randomized to the A Matter of Balance group ($n = 216$) or the control group ($n = 218$). Of these, 388 completed the 6-week follow-up assessment.

- The A Matter of Balance group had significantly better scores ($p < 0.05$) on the Intended Activity and the Mobility Control domains of the Sickness Impact Profile compared to the control group (Table 2.1).
- Data for those considered compliant (completed <u>five or more</u> sessions, $n = 137$) were further evaluated. Compliant A Matter of Balance participants had significantly better falls efficacy, perceived fall management, and Mobility Control domain of the Sickness Impact Profile compared to the control group ($p < 0.05$; Table 2.1).
- The authors also indicated significant improvement at the $p < 0.075$ level in the Sickness Impact Profile total score (Table 2.1) and the Sickness Impact Profile Physical score.
- At the 12-month follow-up, those who were compliant maintained significantly improved scores over the control group in falls efficacy, perceived fall management, and the Sickness Impact Profile total score.

Table 2.1. MEAN CHANGE SCORES FROM BASELINE TO 6-WEEK FOLLOW-UP

Outcome Measure or Construct	Control Group ($n = 190$)	A Matter of Balance ($n = 198$)	Compliant with A Matter of Balance ($n = 131$)	Effect Size at 6-Week Follow-Up (Based on Compliant Data)
Falls efficacy (score range 1–4)	–0.04	0.12	0.15**	0.20
Perceived fall management (score range 1–4)	0.12	0.25	0.37***	0.51
Intended activity (score range 1–4)	–0.02	0.09*	0.09+	—
Sickness Impact Profile total score (score range 1–100)	0.60	–2.52+	–2.63+	0.13 (Mobility Control domain)

+$p < 0.075$, *$p < 0.05$, **$p < 0.01$, ***$p < 0.001$.

Criticisms and Limitations: The control condition was not matched for activity or dose. Multiple assessments—perceived control over falling, perceived ability to manage falls, and intended activity—were developed for the study and not previously validated. Additionally, the authors indicate that the benefits were mostly realized by participants considered to be compliant; those who were compliant may be significantly different from those who dropped out or who were not compliant. Findings may not be generalizable to adults outside of the geographic area or who are not living in senior housing.

Other Relevant Studies and Information:

- A cognitive-behavioral therapy intervention was delivered to adults $\geq$60 years old weekly for 8 weeks (with a 6-month booster) and led to improvements in falls self-efficacy and fear of falling (Parry et al., 2016).
- Eight weeks of Tai Chi Chuan (TCC) was tested for "less robust" older people. The TCC group showed improvements in balance, flexibility, and fear of falling compared to the control group (Zhang et al., 2006).
- A 12-week yoga intervention for older adults decreased fear of falling by 6% and improved balance and lower-body flexibility (Schmid et al., 2010).

Summary and Implications: The A Matter of Balance intervention, a group-based eight-session intervention aimed at reducing fear of falling among older adults in senior housing, was associated with significantly improved "intended activity" and mobility control versus those assigned to a social contact control condition.

CLINICAL CASE: A CLIENT WITH FEAR OF FALLING

Case History
Francisco (he/him), a 77-year-old male of Mexican American descent, attends his first occupational therapy visit after a hip replacement. He is a Marine and is being treated at the Veterans Affairs hospital. He was walking in his neighborhood, crossing through a back alleyway, at the time of the fall that led to his injury. He laid on the ground waiting nearly 20 hours for help. He reported severe pain from the event and revealed he thought he was going to die waiting for assistance. When the occupational therapist (OT) asks, "Are you afraid of falling?" he responds with "I am a Marine. I am not afraid of anything." He mentions that he has stopped going for his daily walks but does not give a reason for this activity restriction. How should the OT proceed?

Suggested Answer
Collectively, the "machismo" of Francisco's culture and his military history likely contribute to his hesitancy to discuss his fears and other feelings. He indirectly reported fear of death as a result of his fall (waiting on the ground for nearly a full day). Although not overtly stated, his activity restriction is

likely a manifestation of his fear of falling. He may believe that avoiding the activity that led to his fall will reduce his risk of falling again, but this only places him at greater risk. Asking about "worry" or "concern" may be more helpful than asking about "fear." Using a standardized assessment to evaluate fear of falling or falls self-efficacy may also provide additional information regarding the client's issues around falls. Addressing behaviors and attitudes related to fall prevention and fear of falling may improve therapy adherence and reduce the risk of a future fall. The OT may want to consider referring the patient to the A Matter of Balance program offered in his community to assist him in regaining falls self-efficacy and returning to his daily activity routine.

References

Parry, S. W., Bamford, C., Deary, V., Finch, T. L., Gray, J., MacDonald, C., McMeekin, P., Sabin, N. J., Steen, I. N., Whitney, S. L., & McColl, E. M. (2016). Cognitive behavioural therapy–based intervention to reduce fear of falling in older people: Therapy development and randomised controlled trial the Strategies for Increasing Independence, Confidence and Energy (STRIDE) study. *Health Technology Assessment, 20*(56). https://doi.org/10.3310/hta20560

Schmid, A. A., Van Puymbroeck, M., & Koceja, D. M. (2010). Effect of a 12-week yoga intervention on fear of falling and balance in older adults: A pilot study. *Archives of Physical Medicine and Rehabilitation, 91*(4), 576–583.

Zhang, J. G., Ishikawa-Takata, K., Yamazaki, H., Morita, T., & Ohta, T. (2006). The effects of Tai Chi Chuan on physiological function and fear of falling in the less robust elderly: An intervention study for preventing falls. *Archives of Gerontology and Geriatrics, 42*(2), 107–116.

3

Combined Occupational Therapy and Medical Approach to Fall Prevention

STACEY L. SCHEPENS NIEMIEC AND RAFAEL WAGAS

PROFET trial

This controlled study has shown the efficacy of a structured interdisciplinary [geriatric medicine and occupational therapy] approach to the management and prevention of falls in older people in a routine service setting. The numbers of subsequent falls and people with recurrent falls were significantly and substantially reduced.

> CLOSE, J., ELLIS, M., HOOPER, R., GLUCKSMAN, E., JACKSON, S., & SWIFT, C. (1999). Prevention of falls in the elderly trial (PROFET): A randomised controlled trial. *The Lancet*, 353(9147), 93–97.

Original Paper: https://doi.org/10.1016/S0140-6736(98)06119-4

Research Question: What are the effects on the outcome and rate of future falls of a structured bidisciplinary assessment of community-dwelling older adults who attend an emergency department with a primary diagnosis of a fall?

Funding: South Thames National Health Service research and development project grant.

Year Study Began: 1995

Year Study Published: 1999

Study Location: United Kingdom

Who Was Studied: Community-dwelling older adult patients (65+ years) who visited the emergency room due to a fall.

Who Was Excluded: Individuals with cognitive impairments defined by an Abbreviated Mental Test score <7 and with no regular caregiver; adults who were not local or spoke little to no English.

How Many Patients: 397

Study Overview: See Figure 3.1.

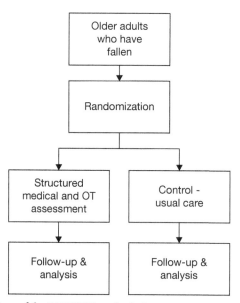

Figure 3.1. Overview of the PROFET study design.

Study Intervention: The intervention group underwent detailed medical and occupational therapy (OT) assessments with corresponding referrals to services as indicated. The medical assessment was comprised of a comprehensive general examination with additional focus on vision, balance, and cognition. Recommendations and referrals were made according to baseline information, fall risk factors, and the primary cause for the index fall. OT assessments took place in the home, following the medical assessment. This visit included a functional evaluation, an environmental assessment, and administration of the Falls Handicap Inventory. Client education inclusive of home modifications was provided along with relevant referrals to community services.

The control group received routine emergency department services, which did not include the focused medical or OT assessments.

Both groups were given monthly falls diary sheets to document falls over a 12-month period.

Follow-Up: Self-report questionnaires were mailed every 4 months for 1 year after the index fall.

Endpoints:

Primary outcomes:

- Falls in 12 months, as measured by self-report questionnaire.
- Functional status, as measured by Barthel Index.

Secondary outcomes:

- Ability to go out alone, as measured by self-report questionnaire.
- Fall-related injury, as measured by self-report questionnaire.
- Hospital admission, as measured by hospital admission data.

RESULTS

- At recruitment, 1031 individuals were eligible; 634 were not enrolled due to ineligibility, refusal of consent, or loss of contact; 397 were randomized to the intervention group ($n = 184$) and the control group ($n = 213$). After the 12-month follow-up, 141 and 163 were included in analysis, respectively.
- After 12 months, median and cumulative number of falls were significantly fewer in the intervention group than in the control group.

- Risk of falling (odds ratio 0.39; 95% confidence interval 0.23–0.6), recurrent falling (0.33; 0.16–0.68), and hospital admission (0.61; 0.35–1.05) across the 12-month period were lower in the intervention group than the control group.
- Barthel scores as a measure of functional status were significantly different between groups and over time, such that the intervention group experienced less decline over time. Additional functional and fall-related outcomes are presented in Table 3.1.

Table 3.1. BETWEEN-GROUP COMPARISONS OF FUNCTIONAL AND FALL-RELATED OUTCOMES FROM BASELINE TO 12 MONTHS

	Control Baseline ($n = 213$)	12 Months ($n = 163$)	Intervention Baseline ($n = 184$)	12 Months ($n = 141$)	p
Barthel Index score ($M \pm SD$)	18.7 ± 2.1	17.3 ± 3.7	19 ± 1.6	18.6 ± 2.5	0.017[a] <0.0001[b]
Reported a fall (n)	141 (66%) (in previous year)	111 (52%)	118 (64%) (in previous year)	59 (32%)	NR
Able to go out alone after fall (n)	168 (79%)	106 (65%)	146 (80%)	108 (77%)	0.04[c]
Reported serious fall-related injury (n)	79 (37%)	16 (8%)	70 (38%)	8 (4%)	0.26[c]
Hospitalization (n)	79 (37%)	97	70 (38%)	69	0.78[c]

NR = not reported.
[a]Group-by-time interaction.
[b]Main effect for time.
[c]Between-group comparison at 12 months.

Criticisms and Limitations: A single physician conducted all medical assessments, whereas multiple occupational therapists were involved in the home assessment component. Length of time to conduct the medical and OT assessments post-fall varied, which may have affected participants' report of fall event details and functional status at baseline. A primary attributable cause to the index fall was unidentified for 28% of the intervention group, which may have been resolved through communication with participants' general practitioner.

Other Relevant Studies and Information:

- Additional studies demonstrate that a multidisciplinary approach to fall prevention that includes occupational therapists as part of the team has proven effective in mitigating fall risk (Davison et al., 2005; Fairhall et al., 2014) and reducing fall rates (Gillespie et al., 2015).
- A Cochrane review demonstrated that home safety interventions for individuals with high risk of falling are most effective when led by occupational therapists versus other personnel such as nurses, community health workers, and domiciliary support workers (Gillespie et al., 2015).
- OT interventions offer benefits in assessing and intervening on the psychological factors relevant to falls (e.g., fear of falling, falls self-efficacy) (Schepens et al., 2012).

Summary and Implications: A structured bidisciplinary approach to falls management and prevention—one that included a comprehensive medical assessment and OT home assessment and intervention—as part of routine clinical services was effective in improving functional and falls outcomes in older adults who have experienced falls. Because the tested approach was designed for integration into routine clinical care, it holds promise as a practical and economical means of addressing the burgeoning challenges of falls in older adults. This study also demonstrates the unique value OT brings to the interdisciplinary team within the fall prevention arena.

CLINICAL CASE: FALL PREVENTION IN ROUTINE CLINICAL CARE

Case History

Earl (he/him), a 69-year-old male with a history of recurrent injurious falls, was assisted by his daughter to the emergency room (ER) following a fall onto an outstretched hand, with resultant shoulder and neck pain. Due to the high frequency of ER visits in the previous 3 months, he is referred to a primary care team to discuss an interdisciplinary approach to his condition. You are a new hire, joining this primary care team as the first occupational therapist member. During rounds, the team strategizes about the patient's plan of care. The group asks for your perspective on how to address the functional limitations of his arm, without realizing the ways OT can participate in addressing this patient's needs post-fall. With your knowledge of the PROFET trial, what would you say to educate the team about OT's role in addressing this patient's fall risk and reducing hospital readmission? What would you recommend for OT's portion of the plan of care?

Suggested Answer

The PROFET trial showed that a structured bidisciplinary approach inclusive of a comprehensive medical exam and home-based OT assessment, with follow-through on recommendations and referrals, improved functional status and decreased subsequent falls in community-dwelling older adults with a primary diagnosis of a fall. As shown in the study, it is important that the medical team gathers a detailed history of falls as well as health and function (e.g., visual acuity, balance, cognition) to accurately identify the cause of the index fall. The OT practitioner can build upon the case by providing a comprehensive home and functional assessment, focusing on environmental hazards and the psychological consequences of falls. OT's intervention for this patient can range from education about home safety and environmental modifications to recommendation for equipment and referral to social services. As demonstrated in the PROFET trial and other studies, the inclusion of the OT discipline on this primary care team could lead to improvements in the patient's functional performance and community mobility and in turn reduce his recurrence of falls and hospitalizations.

References

Davison, J., Bond, J., Dawson, P., Steen, I. N., & Kenny, R. A. (2005). Patients with recurrent falls attending Accident & Emergency benefit from multifactorial intervention—A randomised controlled trial. *Age and Ageing, 34*(2), 162–168. https://doi.org/10.1093/ageing/afi053

Fairhall, N., Sherrington, C., Lord, S. R., Kurrle, S. E., Langron, C., Lockwood, K., Monaghan, N., Aggar, C., & Cameron, I. D. (2014). Effect of a multifactorial, interdisciplinary intervention on risk factors for falls and fall rate in frail older people: A randomised controlled trial. *Age and Ageing, 43*(5), 616–622. https://doi.org/10.1093/ageing/aft204

Gillespie, L. D., Robertson, M. C., Gillespie, W. J., Sherrington, C., Gates, S., Clemson, L. M., & Lamb, S. E. (2015). Interventions for preventing falls in older people living in the community. *Cochrane Database of Systematic Reviews, 2012*(9), Article CD007146. https://doi.org/10.1002/14651858.CD007146.pub3

Schepens, S., Sen, A., Painter, J. A., & Murphy, S. L. (2012). Relationship between fall-related efficacy and activity engagement in community-dwelling older adults: A meta-analytic review. *American Journal of Occupational Therapy, 66*(2), 137–148.

4

Effectiveness of Assistive Technology and Environmental Interventions in Maintaining Independence and Reducing Home Care Costs for the Frail Elderly

SAJAY ARTHANAT

Low-cost assistive technology and environmental interventions may prevent and postpone morbidity.

MANN, W. C., OTTENBACHER, K. J., FRAAS, L., TOMITA, M., & GRANGER, C. V. (1999). Effectiveness of assistive technology and environmental interventions in maintaining independence and reducing home care costs for the frail elderly: A randomized controlled trial. *Archives of Family Medicine, 8*(3), 210–217.

Research Question: Is there a significant difference in functional independence and overall cost of health-related services between frail elderly receiving standard care (control group) and those receiving intensive assistive technology (AT) and environmental interventions (EIs) (treatment group)?

Funding: National Institute on Disability and Rehabilitation Research of the Department of Education, Washington, DC (grant H133E60006); Administration on Aging of the Department of Health and Human Services; and the Andrus Foundation of the American Association of Retired Persons, Washington, DC.

Year Study Began: Not available

Year Study Published: 1999

Study Location: University at Buffalo, Buffalo, NY

Who Was Studied: Physically frail older adults in western New York who were receiving health and rehabilitation services through Medicare–Medicaid. Participants were referred from the 1) Community Alternative Systems Agency of the county, 2) HOSPITAL-based physical medicine rehabilitation programs, and 3) the Visiting Nursing Association.

Who Was Excluded: Individuals with Mini-Mental State Examination (MMSE) score below 23 were excluded.

How Many Patients: 104

Study Overview: See Figure 4.1.

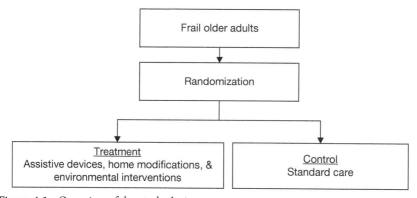

Figure 4.1. Overview of the study design.

Study Intervention: The control group received continuing standard care through home-based senior services. These services varied and included medically directed services following hospitalization and rehabilitation, nursing-directed home care, and non-medical services through the Office for Aging agencies such as Meals-on-Wheels and assistance for instrumental activities of daily living (IADL).

For the treatment group, the study intervention included a comprehensive functional assessment of the person and the home by an occupational therapist, followed by recommendations for needed AT devices and home modifications or EIs, training in the use of devices, and continued follow-up assessment and provision of additional devices and home modifications as needs changed. The occupational therapist was assisted by a nurse and technician experienced in home modifications. Standard care services were also available.

Follow-Up: Participants were assessed with outcome measures every 6 months for 18 months from the initial intervention.

Endpoints:

Primary outcomes:

- Functional Independence Measure (FIM) with both motor and cognitive scores.
- Older Americans Research and Services Center Instrument to measure the impact of service programs on the functional status of older adults.
- Craig Handicap Assessment and Reporting Technique (CHART), a self-reported measure with four subsections—physical independence, mobility, occupation, and social integration.

Secondary outcomes:

- Pain, assessed with the Functional Status Index (FSI).
- Healthcare costs for AT-EIs, in-home personnel, and hospitalization and nursing home care.

RESULTS

- The treatment and control groups were equivalent on all outcome measures at the beginning of the study and were not significantly different demographically.
- After 18 months of intervention:
  - Participants in the treatment group received a mean of 14.2 assistive devices from the study team and a mean of 1.0 device from other sources compared to a mean of 1.9 assistive devices by the control group participants.
  - Participants in the treatment group received a mean of 1.44 EIs from the study team, whereas those in the control group received 0.19 EIs from other sources.

- Participants in both treatment and control groups had declined significantly on IADL total, the FIM (total, motor, and cognitive scores), the MMSE, CHART mobility, and CHART social integration. However, the control group declined significantly more on all outcomes compared to the treatment group (Table 4.1).
- The control group also showed significant declines in FSI pain score, CHART physical independence, and CHART occupation, while the treatment group did not show a significant decline on these measures (Table 4.1).
- The control group had significantly higher costs for institutional care and nurse and case manager visits than the treatment group.

Table 4.1. DIFFERENCES IN TREATMENT AND CONTROL GROUP ON OUTCOME MEASURES FROM BASELINE TO 18 MONTHS

Outcome Measure	Group	Difference from Baseline to 18 Months[a] t (p)	Effect Size
IADL total	Treatment	2.31 (0.03)	0.53
	Control	3.23 (0.002)	0.72
FIM Motor score	Treatment	2.12 (0.04)	0.44
	Control	4.28 (<0.001)	1.00
FIM Cognitive score	Treatment	5.46 (<0.001)	1.20
	Control	3.15 (0.003)	0.74
FIM total	Treatment	3.19 (0.003)	0.69
	Control	4.21 (0.001)	1.02
MMSE	Treatment	2.54 (0.02)	0.49
	Control	2.44 (0.02)	0.61
FSI Pain	Treatment	0.03 (0.98)	0.01
	Control	2.05 (0.05)	0.47
CHART: Physical Independence	Treatment	0.19 (0.85)	0.04
	Control	2.11 (0.04)	0.46
CHART: Mobility	Treatment	1.91 (0.06)	0.39
	Control	2.02 (0.05)	0.45
CHART: Occupation	Treatment	0.60 (0.55)	0.12
	Control	2.15 (0.04)	0.47
CHART: Social Integration	Treatment	2.15 (0.04)	0.45
	Control	3.20 (0.003)	0.70

[a]Higher number indicates greater decline in outcome measures.

Criticisms and Limitations:

- The analysis of the data only included the initial and 18-month follow-up data points. It is unclear why the researchers have not accounted for the data collected in 6-month intervals. A mixed design examining group–time interactions through 6-month intervals would have been appropriate with the given design of the study.

Other Relevant Studies and Information:

- Carnemolla & Bridge (2019) examined self-reported care data from 157 community care recipients (average age 72 years) in Australia who had received home modifications within the past 6 months. A follow-up comparison indicated that home modifications reduced required hours of care by 42% each week.
- Orellano-Colón et al. (2017) developed and tested a culturally sensitive AT implementation program in Puerto Rico for 27 Hispanic adults aged 70 years and older using a mixed methods design. Combined with an ecological validity model, the input from older adults indicated that the program was effective at tailoring the intervention to the needs and circumstances of community-living older people.
- De-Rosende-Celeiro et al. (2019) examined the relationship between the use of assistive products and independence with transfers in the bathroom as well as the role of environmental factors in predicting the implementation of bathroom adaptations. Data gathered from 193 community-dwelling older adults with disabilities showed that the number of categories of assistive products used in the transfer to shower/bath was positively associated with the independent transfer. Social functioning was significantly associated with the implementation of a bathroom adaptation.

Summary and Implications:

- The study demonstrated that a comprehensive approach to implementing low-cost assistive devices and home modifications to support community living of frail older adults may prevent and postpone functional decline among frail older adults living in the community.

CLINICAL CASE: AT AND HOME AUTOMATION INTERVENTION FOR INDIVIDUALS WITH PARKINSON'S DISEASE

Case History

Ernest (he/him), a 77-year-old man with Parkinson's disease, assessed to have postural instability and bilateral involvement of motor symptoms, lives alone in an "in-law" apartment attached to his daughter's house. He has no cognitive symptoms (with MMSE score >24) and is independent in most activities of daily living, with mild assistance of his daughter needed for transfers to and from toilet and bed. He has a history of falls and requires ongoing assistance with IADL including meal preparation and laundry. He recently experienced a fall from his bed and was unable to get up or seek help until his daughter arrived to check on him. Ernest's daughter, who is the primary caregiver, works full time and is therefore concerned that she cannot monitor her father. How should an occupational therapist intervene based on the AT-EI protocol described in the study?

Suggested Answer

The occupational therapist interviewed the client, his daughter, and conducted a comprehensive home safety assessment. Subsequently, a goal attainment scale (GAS) was used to set goals on fall prevention, meal preparation, alerting, and wellness activities. To address these goals, various low-cost commercially available assistive devices combined with home automation devices were installed and paired to the daughter's smartphone. Training on the setup and use was provided to the daughter. The devices included a walker, a raised toilet seat, adaptive devices for cooking, home monitoring cameras at the entry and stairway, motion sensor–activated smart lights in the bedroom and bathroom at night, and a watch with fall detection sensor and fitness tracking. In addition, a grab rail was attached to the bed to ensure safe transfers. A 3-month follow-up assessment indicated that the client met four out of the five goals outlined in the GAS.

References

Carnemolla, P., & Bridge, C. (2019). Housing design and community care: How home modifications reduce care needs of older people and people with disability. *International Journal of Environmental Research and Public Health, 16*(11), Article 1951. https://doi.org/10.3390/ijerph16111951

De-Rosende-Celeiro, I., Torres, G., Seoane-Bouzas, M., & Ávila, A. (2019). Exploring the use of assistive products to promote functional independence in self-care activities in the bathroom. *PLoS One, 14*(4), Article e0215002. https://doi.org/10.1371/journal.pone.0215002

Orellano-Colón, E. M., Morales, F. M., Sotelo, Z., Picado, N., Castro, E. J., Torres, M., Rivero, M., Varas, N., & Jutai, J. (2017). Development of an assistive technology intervention for community older adults. *Physical & Occupational Therapy in Geriatrics, 35*(2), 49–66. https://doi.org/10.1080/02703181.2017.1283656

5

Community Aging in Place, Advancing Better Living for Elders (CAPABLE)

A Bio–Behavioral–Environmental Intervention to Improve Function and Health-Related Quality of Life in Disabled Older Adults

BETH FIELDS

CAPABLE Intervention

> The findings from this study suggest the potential power of a multicomponent intervention that integrates home repair, nursing, and occupational therapy to improve daily function and well-being.
>
> Szanton, S. L., Thorpe, R. J., Boyd, C., Tanner, E. K., Leff, B., Agree, E., Xue, Q.-L., Allen, J. K., Seplaki, C. L., Weiss, C. O., Guralnik, J. M., & Gitlin, L. N. (2011). Community aging in place, advancing better living for elders: A bio-behavioral-environmental intervention to improve function and health-related quality of life in disabled older adults. *Journal of the American Geriatrics Society,* 59(12), 2314–2320.

Original Paper: https://doi.org/10.1111/j.1532-5415.2011.03698.x

Research Question: How does the CAPABLE intervention that targets individual and environmental disability factors in a population of underrepresented and underresourced older adults compare with an attention-control condition in affecting activities of daily living (ADLs) and instrumental ADLs (IADLs) difficulty, health-related quality of life, and falls efficacy?

Funding: The National Institutes of Health, the Claire M. Fagin Fellowship of the Building Academic Geriatric Nursing Capacity Initiative of the John A. Hartford Foundation, the National Institute on Aging, the Paul Beeson Career Development Award Program, the American Federation of Aging Research, Atlantic Philanthropies, the Starr Foundation, and an anonymous donor.

Year Study Began: Not available

Year Study Published: 2011

Study Location: Baltimore, MD

Who Was Studied: Adults aged 65 years or older who were cognitively intact, had low income, and had disability in ADLs.
- 95% female
- 79% African American
- 44% reported difficulty with three or more ADLs

Who Was Excluded: Older adults who were:
- Hospitalized more than three times in the previous year
- Currently receiving in-home rehabilitation
- Diagnosed with a terminal illness with less than 1 year of expected survival
- Planning to move in less than 1 year

How Many Patients: 40

Study Overview: See Figure 5.1.

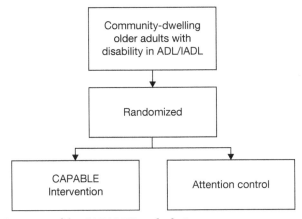

Figure 5.1. Overview of the CAPABLE study design.

Study Intervention: Participants in the CAPABLE intervention group were provided assessment, education, and interactive problem-solving by an interprofessional team consisting of an occupational therapist, a registered nurse, and a handy worker to help the individual achieve self-identified goals targeting daily limitations and associated environmental barriers. Participants received up to six 1-hour home visits with the occupational therapist; up to four 1-hour home visits with the nurse; and as many visits from a handyman as needed during a 6-month period. The intervention draws upon patient-centered care and motivational interviewing strategies.

Participants in the attention-control group received up to 10 sessions, lasting 1 hour, with a trained research assistant (not an occupational therapist or nurse) who engaged them in reminiscence and sedentary activities of their choice.

Follow-Up: Participants were tested at baseline and after pilot trial completion 6 months later.

Endpoints:

Primary outcomes:

- Functional impairments in ADL and/or IADL (self-reported level of difficulty).

Secondary outcomes:

- Health-related quality of life (EuroQol-5 Dimension [EQ-5D] or EuroQoL).

- Falls efficacy (self-report of confidence in performing activities without falling).
- Program acceptability questionnaire.

RESULTS

- Forty participants were randomized to the CAPABLE intervention group ($n = 24$) and the attention-control group ($n = 16$). Of these, 35 participants' data were analyzed at 6 months. No between-group differences at baseline in age, sex, education, ADL or IADL difficulty, quality of life, cognition, or falls efficacy were detected (Table 5.1).
- Moderate effect sizes favoring the intervention for differences in mean change between the intervention and control groups from baseline to follow-up were found for ADL and IADL difficulty (Table 5.1).
- Strong and moderate effect sizes favoring the intervention were found for quality of life on the EuroQoL and the EQ-5D, respectively (Table 5.1).
- A moderate effect size favoring the intervention was found for falls efficacy (Table 5.1).
- Participants in the intervention (94%) and control (53%) groups reported that participation in the study made their lives easier.

Table 5.1. COMPARISON OF INTERVENTION AND
CONTROL GROUP PARTICIPANTS

| Outcome Measure | Change Score = Posttest – Pretest Score | | Effect Size[b] |
	CAPABLE Intervention ($n = 24$) Mean ± SD	Attention Control ($n = 16$) Mean ± SD	
Disability ADL difficulty[a]	−1.4 ± 0.4	−0.5 ± 0.9	0.63
IADL difficulty[a]	−1.1 ± 0.1	−0.2 ± 0.8	0.62
Quality of life EuroQoL	17.9 ± 3.7	−0.6 ± 5.8	0.89
EQ-5D	−0.9 ± 0.4	0 ± 0.5	0.48
Falls efficacy[a]	−5 ± 1.4	5.4 ± 10.5	0.55

[a]Lower score indicates improvement.
[b]Mean of change in intervention from pretest to posttest minus mean of control from pretest to posttest divided by pooled standard deviation. Reported effect sizes suggest favorable results for the intervention group.

Criticisms and Limitations: Outcomes relied on self-reported data, which may be subject to recall bias. Analyses were executed on a modified intention-to-treat basis where participants unavailable for follow-up were excluded. Lastly, participants were primarily female and African American; thus, the results may lack generalizability.

Other Relevant Studies and Information:

- A number of larger randomized trials comparing ADL and IADL performance in a primarily female and African American sample have come to similar conclusions after completing the CAPABLE intervention (Szanton et al., 2016, 2019).
- Trials comparing the CAPABLE intervention versus a usual care cohort in low-income participants living in the community have also demonstrated that the CAPABLE intervention is associated with lower health service utilization rates (e.g., hospitalizations, home health, specialty care) and overall Medicaid spending (Spoelstra et al., 2019; Szanton et al., 2018).
- Given the favorable findings associated with the program, CAPABLE has attracted public attention and is being considered for inclusion as a new reimbursable model by the Department of Health & Human Services (Biden, n.d.; Coleman, 2019).

Summary and Implications: A patient-centered, interprofessional team–based intervention for community-dwelling older adults had favorable effects on ADL and IADL functional status, falls efficacy, and quality of life in comparison to a control intervention focused on reminiscence and sedentary activities. Additionally, participants reported acceptability and perceived benefit of the CAPABLE intervention.

CLINICAL CASE: FREQUENT FALLER

Case History

Gloria (she/her), a 68-year-old community-dwelling woman with cardiovascular disease, reports to her care manager through the local Area Agency on Aging (AAA) that she has recently experienced several falls in her home. She refuses to make an appointment and travel to see her primary care provider because her falls have not resulted in any serious injuries. Based on this client's self-report, how should she be approached?

Suggested Answer

The care manager shares an overview of CAPABLE with Gloria and asks whether she would be interested in receiving the home-based, person-centered intervention. The client expresses interest, so the care manager contacts the occupational therapist, nurse, and handy worker contracted through the AAA who have all completed online training to provide CAPABLE (for training information, visit https://learn.nursing.jhu.edu/instruments-interventions/CAPABLE/CAPABLE). After the team has determined the client's eligibility, each professional schedules their visits with the client to help address home environmental barriers, safety concerns, and functional limitations. In the unlikely event that significant functional limitations and safety concerns persist after intervention, the occupational therapist and nurse would discuss with the client how and why to request a referral from her primary care provider for home health services.

References

Biden, J. (2020). *Build back better.* https://www.c-span.org/video/?c4894067/user-clip-joe-bidens-shoutout-capable

Coleman, K. (2019). *Implementing supplemental benefits for chronically ill enrollees.* https://www.cms.gov/Medicare/Health-Plans/HealthPlansGenInfo/Downloads/Supplemental_Benefits_Chronically_Ill_HPMS_042419.pdf

Spoelstra, S. L., Sikorskii, A., Gitlin, L. N., Schueller, M., Kline, M., & Szanton S. L. (2019). Dissemination of the CAPABLE model of care in a Medicaid waiver program to improve physical function. *Journal of American Geriatrics Society, 67*(2), 363–370. https://doi.org/10.1111/jgs.15713

Szanton, S. L., Alfonso, Y. N., Leff, B., Guralnik, J., Wolff, J. L., Stockwell, I., Gitlin, L. N., & Bishai, D. (2018). Medicaid cost savings of a preventive home visit program for disabled older adults. *Journal of American Geriatrics Society, 66*(3), 614–620. https://doi.org/10.1111/jgs.15143

Szanton, S. L., Leff, B., Wolff, J. L., Roberts, L., & Gitlin, L. N. (2016). Home-based care program reduces disability and promotes aging in place. *Health Affairs (Millwood), 35*(9), 1558–1563. https://doi.org/10.1377/hlthaff.2016.0140

Szanton, S. L., Xue, Q. L., Leff, B., Guralnik, J., Wolff, J. L., Tanner, E. K., Boyd, C., Thorpe, R. J., Bishai, D., & Gitlin, L. N. (2019). Effect of a biobehavioral environmental approach on disability among low-income older adults: A randomized clinical trial. *JAMA Internal Medicine, 179*(2), 204–211. https://doi.org/10.1001/jamaintern med.2018.6026

6

Occupational Therapy for Independent-Living Older Adults

STACEY L. SCHEPENS NIEMIEC, ELISSA S. LEE, AND
ELIZABETH A. PYATAK

[T]his study provided a rigorous test of the relative effectiveness of a
nonprofessionally led activity group (the social control group) and a
professionally designed program based on OT principles. Because both
programs involved subjects with activity, our findings call into question
the cliché that "keeping busy keeps you healthy."
CLARK, F., AZEN, S. P., ZEMKE, R., JACKSON, J., CARLSON, M., MANDEL,
D., HAY, J., JOSEPHSON, K., CHERRY, B., HESSEL, C., PALMER, J., &
LIPSON, L. (1997). Occupational therapy for independent-living older adults:
A randomized controlled trial. *The Journal of the American Medical Association*,
278(16), 1321–1326.

Original Paper: https://doi.org/10.1001/jama.1997.03550160041036

Research Question: Is preventive occupational therapy (OT) for independent-
living older adults efficacious?

Funding: The National Institute on Aging and the National Center for Medical
Rehabilitation Research at the National Institutes of Health; the Agency
for Health Care Policy and Research; the American Occupational Therapy
Foundation Center at the University of Southern California for the Study of

Occupation and Its Relation to Adaptation; the RGK Foundation; Lumex, Inc.; and Smith & Nephew Rolyan.

Year Study Began: 1994

Year Study Published: 1997

Study Location: Los Angeles, CA

Who Was Studied: Independent-living adults (English- or Mandarin-speaking) aged 60 years or above.
- 47% Asian, 23% White, 17% African American, 11% Hispanic
- 73% lived alone
- 27% reported one disability or more

Who Was Excluded: Older adults unable to live independently or who exhibited marked dementia.

How Many Patients: 361

Study Overview: Study participants were randomized to one of three groups: OT program, social activity program (active-control group), or a non-treatment control group (usual care) (Figure 6.1).

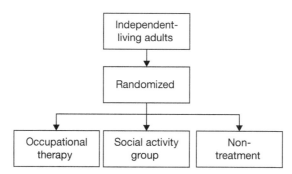

Figure 6.1. Overview of the study design.

Study Intervention: Participants in the OT group were provided with an occupational therapist–led group focused on health through occupation to help participants better appreciate the importance of meaningful activity in their lives, as well as impart specific knowledge about how to select or perform activities to achieve a healthy and meaningful life. Participants received 2 hours per week of group OT and a total of 9 hours of individual therapy during a 9-month treatment period.

There were two control conditions: a non-treatment control (i.e., care as usual with no intervention) and a social activity control. The social control group was facilitated by non-professionals and focused on generalized activities designed to encourage social interaction among group members, such as attending community outings and playing games. These sessions followed a meeting schedule similar to that of the OT group, minus the individualized sessions.

Follow-Up: Participants were tested at baseline, at the end of a 9-month treatment period, and after a 6-month no-treatment follow-up period.

Endpoints:

Primary outcomes:

- Functional impairments in physical and social domains (Functional Status Questionnaire).
- Overall life satisfaction (Life Satisfaction Index-Z).
- Frequency of depressive symptoms (Center for Epidemiologic Studies Depression Scale).
- General health (Medical Outcomes Study Short-Form General Health Survey).
- Overall physical and mental health status (RAND 36-Item Health Status Survey, Short Form [RAND SF-36]).

RESULTS

- Treatment adherence was similar in the OT and social activity-control groups, with OT group participants attending an average of 60% of sessions and social activity control group participants attending an average of 61% of sessions.
- Overall, significant benefits for OT treatment were found across multiple health and quality-of-life domains, including life satisfaction, health perception, and seven of eight scales on the RAND SF-36 (Table 6.1).
- Scores for the social activity-control group were similar to, and in one case significantly worse than,[1] those of the no-treatment control group, and thus were combined in analysis.

---

[1] RAND SF-36 Vitality subscale, $p = 0.007$ between-group difference, $p = 0.04$ after adjusting for baseline differences.

- Within-group analyses of the OT treatment group demonstrate that, compared with other ethnic groups, Asians (non-Mandarin-speaking) exhibited greater improvement on the Life Satisfaction Index-Z, Center for Epidemiologic Studies Depression Scale, and Medical Outcomes Study Health Perception Index, while Hispanics showed greater improvement on the RAND SF-36 General Health subscale.

Table 6.1. BETWEEN-GROUP DIFFERENCES AND CHANGE IN HEALTH-RELATED QUALITY OF LIFE

Measure	Between-Group Difference in Mean Change Scores	Adjusted Between-Group Difference in Mean Change Scores[a]	*p* (One-Tailed)[a]
RAND SF-36 subscales			
Bodily Pain	9.5	6.0	0.03
Physical Functioning	7.0	10.9	0.008
Role Functioning	7.1	13.1	0.02
General Health	2.1	4.4	0.06
Vitality	4.9	7.9	0.004
Social Functioning	4.7	5.3	0.05
Role Emotional	6.6	10.1	0.05
General Mental Health	2.7	5.6	0.02

[a]Adjusted for baseline scores, sex, age group, disability status, and living status as covariates. p values are given for adjusted change scores.

Criticisms and Limitations: The study findings may not generalize to older adults in different living situations (e.g., rural communities, nursing home residents) or of different socioeconomic status.

Other Relevant Studies and Information:

- Companion articles analyzed the cost-effectiveness of the Well Elderly intervention (Hay et al., 2002) as well as the long-term carryover of intervention effects 6 months after completing the intervention (Clark et al., 2001).
- A Well Elderly effectiveness study was implemented in diverse community settings with a sample of older adults at high risk for experiencing health disparities. This was delivered within a shorter time interval (6 months as opposed to 9 months) and with fewer individual

and group sessions and was found to be both effective and cost-effective (Clark et al., 2011).

- Researchers have evaluated interventions based on the Well Elderly study in a variety of contexts, with overall positive findings (Cassidy et al., 2017; Johansson & Björklund, 2016; Matuska et al., 2003; Mountain et al., 2017; Schepens Niemiec et al., 2018; Zilbershlag et al., 2019).

Summary and Implications: A preventive health OT program for independent-living older adults had favorable effects on functional status, quality of life, and life satisfaction, slowing or overriding age-related health declines commonly experienced in later life. These positive results were exclusive to the occupation-based treatment group, demonstrating OT's value beyond non-professionally led social activity engagement. The comprehensive benefits of preventive OT have strong potential to not only improve the quality of life and health of older individuals but also forestall the need for more intensive, costly health services in the future.

CLINICAL CASE: PROMOTING HEALTH OF OLDER LIVING IN AN INDEPENDENT-LIVING COMMUNITY

Case History

An occupational therapist is working at a continuing care retirement community. Recently, the facility has seen a significant increase in residents who require home health and skilled nursing services. The facility director wants to expand their wellness program offerings in place for the independent-living residents, to foster well-being and prevent health declines in a cost-effective way. Presently, residents can attend weekly group sessions, led by an activities coordinator, where they do activities such as crafting, sing-alongs, and bingo. The director has heard that evidence-based approaches to older adult general wellness exist but is unsure of the best option. They look to the occupational therapist for ideas. Using the Well Elderly study and related evidence, how should the occupational therapist respond?

Suggested Answer

The Well Elderly study and others demonstrate that preventive OT for independent-living seniors can promote physical and mental well-being, as well as forestall age-related declines that can lead to a need for medically necessary services. The occupational therapist can educate the director about why the social activity group is not preventing the declines in health they are seeing in the residents—merely keeping residents busy is not health-promoting. Instead, the occupational therapist suggests OT-led group-based sessions combined with individual visits, focusing on health through occupation and selection of activities that contribute to a healthy and meaningful lifestyle in older adulthood.

> A program as such is likely to improve the residents' quality of life and defer the need for more costly services within the facility.

References

Cassidy, T. B., Richards, L. G., & Eakman, A. M. (2017). Feasibility of a Lifestyle Redesign˚–inspired intervention for well older adults. *American Journal of Occupational Therapy*, 71(4). https://doi.org/10.5014/ajot.2017.024430

Clark, F., Azen, S. P., Carlson, M., Mandel, D., Labree, L., Hay, J., Zemke, R., Jackson, J., & Lipson, L. (2001). Embedding health-promoting changes into the daily lives of independent-living older adults: Long-term follow-up of occupational therapy intervention. *The Journals of Gerontology Series B: Psychological Sciences and Social Sciences*, 56(1). https://doi.org/10.1093/geronb/56.1.p60

Clark, F., Jackson, J., Carlson, M., Chou, C.-P., Cherry, B. J., Jordan-Marsh, M., Knight, B. G., Mandel, D., Blanchard, J., Granger, D. A., Wilcox, R. R., Lai, M. Y., White, B., Hay, J., Lam, C., Marterella, A., & Azen, S. P. (2011). Effectiveness of a lifestyle intervention in promoting the well-being of independently living older people: Results of the Well Elderly 2 randomised controlled trial. *Journal of Epidemiology and Community Health*, 66(9), 782–790. https://doi.org/10.1136/jech.2009.099754

Hay, J., Labree, L., Luo, R., Clark, F., Carlson, M., Mandel, D., Zemke, R., Jackson, J., & Azen, S. P. (2002). Cost-effectiveness of preventive occupational therapy for independent-living older adults. *Journal of the American Geriatrics Society*, 50(8), 1381–1388. https://doi.org/10.1046/j.1532-5415.2002.50359.x

Johansson, A., & Björklund, A. (2016). The impact of occupational therapy and lifestyle interventions on older persons' health, well-being, and occupational adaptation: A mixed-design study. *Scandinavian Journal of Occupational Therapy*, 23(3), 207–219.

Maeir, T., Beit-Yosef, A., Wechsler, T., Safra, Y., Zilbershlag, Y., Katz, N., & Gilboa, Y. (2021). The feasibility and efficacy of an Israeli Lifestyle Redesign®–based program for well older adults: A pilot study. *OTJR: Occupation, Participation and Health*, 41(1), 47–55. https://doi.org/10.1177/1539449220928141

Matuska, K., Giles-Heinz, A., Flinn, N., Neighbor, M., & Bass-Haugen, J. (2003). Outcomes of a pilot occupational therapy wellness program for older adults. *American Journal of Occupational Therapy*, 57(2), 220–224.

Mountain, G., Windle, G., Hind, D., Walters, S., Keertharuth, A., Chatters, R., Sprange, K., Craig, C., Cook, S., Lee, E., Chater, T., Woods, R., Newbould, L., Powell, L., Shortland, K., & Roberts, J. (2017). A preventative lifestyle intervention for older adults (Lifestyle Matters): A randomised controlled trial. *Age and Ageing*, 46(4), 627–634. https://doi.org/10.1093/ageing/afx021

Schepens Niemiec, S. L., Blanchard, J., Vigen, C. L., Martínez, J., Guzmán, L., Concha, A., Fluke, M., & Carlson, M. (2018). Evaluation of ¡Vivir Mi Vida! to improve health and wellness of rural-dwelling, late middle-aged Latino adults: Results of a feasibility and pilot study of a lifestyle intervention. *Primary Health Care Research & Development*, 19(5), 448–463.

7

Occupational Therapy for Older Adults with Dementia and Their Caregivers

JENNY MARTÍNEZ

Ten sessions of community occupational therapy over 5 weeks improved the daily functioning of older adults with dementia and the sense of competence among their primary caregivers.

GRAFF, M. J. L., VERNOOIJ-DASSEN, M. J. M., THIJSSEN, M., DEKKER, J., HOEFNAGELS, W. H. L., & OLDERIKKERT, M. G. M. (2006). Community based occupational therapy for patients with dementia and their caregivers: Randomized control trial. *BMJ*, *33*, 1196–1199.

Original Paper: https://doi.org/10.1136/bmj.39001.688843.BE

Research Question: What are the effects of community-based occupational therapy on daily functioning of older adults with dementia and the sense of competence of their caregivers?

Funding: The Dutch Alzheimer Association, the Radboud University Nijmegen Medical Center, and the Dutch Occupational Therapy Association.

Year Study Began: 2001

Year Study Published: 2006

Study Location: the Netherlands

Who Was Studied: Dyads were comprised of community-dwelling adults aged 65 years or above with a diagnosis of mild to moderate dementia and their primary caregiver (must have provided care at least once a week).

Who Was Excluded: Older adults with a score >12 on the Geriatric Depression Scale or severe behavioral or psychological symptoms in dementia; older adults and caregivers with severe illness.

How Many Patients: 135

Study Overview: See Figure 7.1.

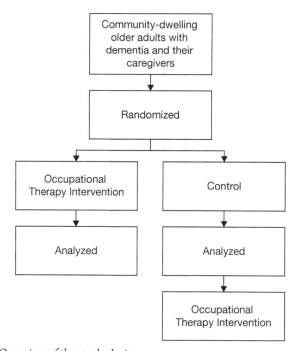

Figure 7.1. Overview of the study design.

Study Intervention: The intervention group received 10 sessions of occupational therapy at home over 5 weeks, each lasting 1 hour. The intervention was delivered by trained occupational therapists experienced in delivering treatment according to a client-centered guideline for older adults with dementia. Treatment focused on the older adult with dementia–caregiver dyad. Dyads defined goals, identified meaningful activities they wanted to improve, and participated in observations of their everyday interactions in the home environment. Dyads were taught ways to optimize compensatory and environmental strategies to improve daily functioning, while caregivers also received further training on skills to sustain performance such as effective supervision, problem-solving, and coping strategies.

The control group did not receive occupational therapy and was stratified by level of dementia (i.e., mild or moderate). The control group received the occupational therapy intervention following completion of the study.

Follow-Up: Older adults with dementia and their caregivers were assessed before the intervention, at 6 weeks (immediately following the intervention period), and at 12 weeks.

Endpoints:

Primary outcomes for older adults with dementia:

- Daily functioning, as measured by the Assessment of Motor and Process Skills (AMPS), in which scores range from –3 to 4 (higher scores are indicative of better process skills).
  - A change over time of 0.5 points was considered clinically relevant.
- Performance in daily activities, as measured by the Interview of Deterioration of Daily Activities in Dementia (IDDD), in which scores range from 0 to 44 (lower scores are indicative of less need for assistance).
  - A 20% improvement was considered clinically relevant.

Primary outcomes for caregivers:

- Overall sense of competence, as measured by the Sense of Competence Questionnaire (SCQ), in which scores range from 27 to 135 (higher scores are indicative of a greater sense of competence).
  - A 5-point difference was considered clinically relevant.

Secondary outcomes for older adults: Comorbidity, depression, cognition, behavior.

Secondary outcomes for caregivers: Depression, relationship with the older adult with dementia.

RESULTS

- Overall, 135 older adults with dementia and their caregivers were randomized to the occupational therapy group ($n = 68$) and the control group ($n = 67$).
- At 6 weeks, participants in the intervention group functioned significantly better in daily life than those in the control group. For intervention versus control, mean process scores obtained by the AMPS process scale were 1.2 (standard deviation [SD] 0.7) versus 0.2 (SD 0.8). Mean performance interview scores as determined via the IDDD were 14.4 (SD 6.1) versus 25.3(SD 8.6).
- At 6 weeks, primary caregivers in the intervention group felt significantly more competent than those in the control group. For intervention versus control, mean competence scores obtained via the SCQ were 104.6 (SD 13.4) versus 88.4 (SD 13.7).
- At 6 weeks, clinically relevant improvement was achieved more frequently by participants in the intervention group for the process outcome as captured via the AMPS. For intervention versus control, 84% versus 9%; and for the performance interview, for intervention versus control, 78% versus 12%.
- At 6 weeks, clinically relevant improvement was achieved more frequently by caregivers in the intervention group for feelings of competence as evaluated by the SCQ (for intervention vs. control, 58% vs. 18%).
- Effect sizes for all primary outcomes were higher than those found in drug trials or other psychosocial interventions for persons with dementia and remained at 12 weeks (effect sizes at 6 weeks = 2.5 [AMPS], 2.3 [IDDD], and 1.2 [SCQ]; at 12 weeks = 2.7 [AMPS], 2.4 [IDDD], and 0.8 [SCQ]).
- At 12 weeks, the daily function of participants as evaluated by the AMPS and the IDDD in the intervention group was significantly better than that of the control group (Table 7.1).

Table 7.1. STUDY RESULTS

Measure	Between-Group Difference in Mean Change Scores at 6 Weeks vs Baseline	Effect Size at 6 Weeks	p (One-Tailed)[a]	Between-Group Difference in Mean Change Scores at 12 Weeks vs Baseline	Effect Size at 12 Weeks	p (One-Tailed)[a]
AMPS process	1.5 (95% CI 1.3–1.7)	2.5	<0.0001	1.6 (95% CI 1.3–1.8)	2.7	<0.0001
IDDD performance	–11.7 (95% CI –13.6 to –9.7)	2.3	<0.0001	–13.6 (95% CI –15.8 to –11.3)	2.4	<0.0001
Caregiver sense of competence	11.0 (95% CI 9.2–12.8)	1.2	<0.0001	9.6 (95% CI 4.7–14.5)	0.8	<0.0001

CI = confidence interval.
[a]Adjusted for age differences as covariates.

Criticisms and Limitations: Occupational therapists and participants were not blinded to treatment allocations; participants were recruited primarily from the outpatient clinics of a university hospital in the Netherlands; thus, findings may not generalize to older adults with mild to moderate dementia outside of this setting.

Other Relevant Studies and Information:

- Subsequent studies support the positive impact of non-pharmacologic interventions such as mindfulness-based approaches and multicomponent interventions on caregiver burden, stress, and subjective well-being (Cheng et al., 2020).
- Evidence and guidelines support non-pharmacologic approaches as the first line of treatment in standard, comprehensive care for persons with dementia (Gitlin et al., 2012).
- Subsequent studies support the positive effects of occupational therapy interventions on behavioral symptoms and functional dependence of older adults with dementia, as well as caregiver well-being (Gitlin et al., 2010, 2018).
- Recent reviews of the literature on the effectiveness of interventions for persons with Alzheimer's disease and their caregivers have found

strong evidence for occupational therapy interventions that a) provided education, support, and training for family members and other informal caregivers (Piersol et al., 2017; Piersol & Jensen, 2017); b) include person-centered, individually tailored, environment-based approaches (Jensen & Padilla, 2017; Piersol & Jensen, 2017); and c) use occupation-based interventions, routine physical exercise, and errorless learning strategies (Piersol & Jensen, 2017; Smallfield & Heckenlaible, 2017).

Summary and Implications: A community-based occupational therapy program for older adults with dementia and their caregivers improved daily functioning in participants and sense of competence in their primary caregivers. Improvements were sustained over 12 weeks. The findings support the implementation of this intervention, the importance of addressing the older adult with dementia–caregiver dyad, and the benefits of occupational therapy in dementia care.

CLINICAL CASE: HOME-BASED OCCUPATIONAL THERAPY FOR DEMENTIA CARE

Case History

Maya (she/her), an 85-year-old woman with Alzheimer's disease, lives in a two-story home with her daughter, who also serves as her primary caregiver. Maya was diagnosed with Alzheimer's disease after increasing difficulty paying bills and keeping track of her daily activities (e.g., dates with friends, doctor's appointments). Maya has been referred by her primary care physician to home-based occupational therapy. Her physician hopes this referral will help promote safety and functional performance at home and provide Maya's daughter with additional support.

Based on the results of this study, how should the occupational therapist proceed?

Suggested Answer

This study showed that community-based occupational therapy for older adults with dementia and their caregivers was beneficial. The older adult with dementia–caregiver dyad benefited from occupational therapy's focus on meaningful activities, defining personally meaningful goals, modifying the home and environment to improve function, and providing targeted training for caregiving-related skills.

The occupational therapist in this case should first complete a comprehensive assessment to understand a) Maya's valued occupations, needs, and goals; b) the primary caregiver's goals; c) Maya's performance of daily activities and caregiving interactions with her daughter; and d) opportunities to modify Maya's home and environment. The program established by the occupational therapist should address the goals and meaningful activities Maya and her daughter identified as priorities. By collaborating with Maya and her daughter, the occupational therapist can also address compensatory and environmental strategies to optimize Maya's performance and safety during everyday tasks. Further training in caregiving skills (e.g., supervision strategies, coping strategies) for Maya's daughter should also be provided to enhance her sense of competence and well-being.

References

Cheng, S. T., Li, K. K., Losada, A., Zhang, F., Au, A., Thompson, L. W., & Gallagher-Thompson, D. (2020). The effectiveness of nonpharmacological interventions for informal dementia caregivers: An updated systematic review and meta-analysis. *Psychology and Aging, 35*(1), 55–77.

Gitlin, L. N., Arthur, P., Piersol, C., Hessels, V., Wu, S. S., Dai, Y., & Mann, W. C. (2018). Targeting behavioral symptoms and functional decline in dementia: A randomized clinical trial. *Journal of the American Geriatrics Society, 66,* 339–345. https://doi.org/10.1111/jgs.15194

Gitlin, L. N., Kales, H. C., & Lyketsos, C. G. (2012). Nonpharmacologic management of behavioral symptoms in dementia. *Journal of the American Medical Association, 308*(19), 2020–2029. https://doi.org/10.1001/jama.2012.36918

Gitlin, L. N., Winter, L., Dennis, M. P., Hodgson, N., & Hauck, W. W. (2010). Targeting and managing behavioral symptoms in individuals with dementia: A randomized trial of a nonpharmacological intervention. *Journal of the American Geriatrics Society, 58,* 1465–1474. https://doi.org/10.1111/j.1532-5415.2010.02971.x

Jensen, L., & Padilla, R. (2017). Effectiveness of environment-based interventions that address behavior, perception, and falls in people with Alzheimer's disease and related major neurocognitive disorders: A systematic review. *American Journal of Occupational Therapy, 71,* Article 7105180030. https://doi.org/10.5014/ajot.2017.027409

Piersol, C. V., Canton, K., Connor, S. E., Giller, I., Lipman, S., & Sager, S. (2017). Effectiveness of interventions for caregivers of people with Alzheimer's disease and related major neurocognitive disorders: A systematic review. *American Journal of Occupational Therapy, 71,* Article 7105180020. https://doi.org/10.5014/ajot.2017.027581

Piersol, C. V., & Jensen, L. (2017). *Occupational therapy practice guidelines for adults with Alzheimer's disease and related major neurocognitive disorders.* AOTA Press.

Smallfield, S., & Heckenlaible, C. (2017). Effectiveness of occupational therapy interventions to enhance occupational performance for adults with Alzheimer's disease and related major neurocognitive disorders: A systematic review. *American Journal of Occupational Therapy, 71,* Article 7105180010. https://doi.org/10.5014/ajot.2017.024752

8

Individualized Activity-Based Interventions for People with Dementia and Informal Caregivers

PREETHY S. SAMUEL

TAP (Tailored Activity Program)

> This study identifies a process for customizing activities to abilities and training families in use of activities in daily care.
> GITLIN, L. N., WINTER, L., BURKE, J., CHERNETT, N., DENNIS, M. P., & HAUCK, W. W. (2008). Tailored activities to manage neuropsychiatric behaviors in persons with dementia and reduce caregiver burden: A randomized pilot study. *The American Journal of Geriatric Psychiatry, 16*(3), 229–239.

Original Paper: https://doi.org/10.1097/JGP.0b013e318160da72

Research Question: Can an activity-based intervention decrease behavioral challenges of people with dementia and reduce caregiver burden?

Funding: The National Institute of Mental Health

Year Study Began: 2005

Year Study Published: 2008

Study Location: Philadelphia, PA

Who Was Studied: Community-dwelling older adults with moderate-stage dementia who could participate in two or more activities of daily living and co-resident caregivers who provided ≥4 hours of daily care and were willing to learn activity use.

Who Was Excluded: People with dementia who were unresponsive or were bed-/chair-bound for ≥22 hours/day or had other major diagnoses (e.g., schizophrenia, active cancer, terminal illness) were excluded.

Caregivers seeking nursing home placement or involved in another study were excluded.

How Many Patients: 60 dyads of individuals and caregivers

Study Overview: See Figure 8.1.

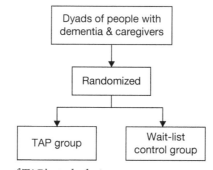

Figure 8.1. Overview of TAP's study design.

Study Intervention: Eight TAP sessions were implemented over 4 months via six 90-minute home visits and two 15-minute telephone calls. In the first two in-home sessions, occupational therapists used activity-based assessments and interviewing to discern daily challenges, routines, and interests. Therapists developed activity prescriptions for three activities ranging in complexity such as making salad (multistep), playing catch with a grandchild (one or two steps), and listening to music (sensory-based) that were introduced in the subsequent sessions through direct demonstrations. Caregivers were taught stress-reducing techniques and how to downgrade activities to prepare for future declines in capability. The wait-list control group received the same intervention at the end of the study period.

Follow-Up: 4 months

Endpoints: The primary outcome of the TAP was to decrease behavioral challenges of individuals with dementia. They also evaluated depression, activity engagement, and quality of life of the person with dementia. The caregiver outcomes were burden (subjective and objective), depression, mastery, confidence, and skill enhancement in managing activity-related tasks.

RESULTS

- 84 dyads screened (19 dyads ineligible, 5 unwilling to participate) → 60 dyads randomized to treatment or wait-list control group → 4 dyads at 4-month follow-up (3 in treatment group, 1 in control group).
- Average cost of activity-related materials (e.g., games, beads, organizers) per dyad was about $70.
- Beneficial treatment outcomes for people with dementia:
  - Reduced frequency of behavioral problems ($p = 0.009$, Cohen's $d = 0.72$; Table 8.1), specifically shadowing ($p = 0.003$, Cohen's $d = 3.10$), repetitive questioning ($p = 0.023$, Cohen's $d = 1.22$), agitation ($p = 0.014$, Cohen's $d = 0.75$), and argumentativeness ($p = 0.010$, Cohen's $d = 0.77$).
  - Greater engagement in activities ($p = 0.029$, Cohen's $d = 0.61$; Table 8.1) and ability to keep busy ($p = 0.017$, Cohen's $d = 0.71$; Table 8.1) compared to control group.
- Beneficial treatment outcomes for caregivers:
  - Decreased caregiver burden: a) ~1-hour reduction in time spent doing things to help care recipients, whereas control group showed a 2-hour increase and b) ~5-hour decrease in "on-duty hours," whereas the control group showed a 2-hour increase.
  - Increased skill level in activity use with care recipients: a) greater confidence in using activities, b) increased mastery, and c) better use of task simplification strategies.
  - Treatment outcomes were not moderated by caregivers' depressive symptoms at baseline; the intervention benefited all caregivers regardless of initial depressive symptoms.

- Overall acceptability of the TAP was good:
  - All participants with dementia across groups were *very engaged* (70%) or *somewhat engaged* (20%) in activities with interventionists. Most showed *a lot of pleasure* (67%) or *some pleasure* (30%) in activities. Only ~7% of participants refused participation, and 2% were agitated in a treatment session.
  - Most (85%) caregivers found the intervention to be very useful and demonstrated good understanding of strategies.

Table 8.1. INTERVENTION OUTCOMES FOR CARE RECIPIENTS AND CAREGIVERS

Outcomes	TAP group		Control group		Difference	
	Baseline M (SD)	4 Months M (SD)	Baseline M (SD)	4 Months M (SD)	p	d
Care recipient						
Behavior problems frequency	30.5 (30.3)	18.8 (17.6)	41.5 (70.5)	60.8 (85.3)	0.009	0.72
Activity engagement	2.1 (0.4)	2.3 (0.3)	1.9 (0.4)	2.0 (0.4)	−0.029	0.61
Able to keep busy	1.6 (0.9)	2.2 (0.7)	1.7 (0.8)	1.6 (0.9)	0.017	0.71
Caregiver						
Objective burden[a]						
Helping care recipient (hours)	6.3 (4.3)	5.4 (2.5)	6.2 (3.3)	8.6 (5.7)	0.005	1.14
Felt like on duty (hours)	18.2 (7.3)	13.4 (7.6)	15.5 (7.7)	17.6 (7.1)	0.001	1.01
Skill[b]						
Mastery	3.4 (0.5)	3.7 (0.6)	3.7 (0.6)	3.7 (0.6)	0.013	0.55
Task simplification strategies	3.0 (0.6)	3.2 (0.5)	2.8 (0.5)	2.9 (0.6)	0.023	0.71

[a]Lower values represent favorable outcomes.
[b]Higher values represent favorable outcomes.

Criticisms and Limitations: Key limitations include a small sample size and potentially biased caregiver-reported outcomes. Cost, time-intensive intervention, lack of clarity on replication, and standardization of training therapists on this approach may limit TAP's dissemination.

Other Relevant Studies and Information:

- Ongoing research indicates that the TAP is cost-effective (Gitlin, Hodgson et al., 2010; Gitlin, Winter et al., 2010), is useful for veterans with dementia (Gitlin et al., 2013, 2018), and can be modified for international use such as in Brazil (Novelli et al., 2018) and Australia (O'Connor et al., 2014).
- Evidence from larger community-based research studies on the effectiveness of individualized home-based occupational therapy for people with dementia is mixed (Döpp et al., 2015; Graff et al., 2006, 2008).
- Other strategies to improve the quality of life of family caregivers include training them to safely assist their care recipients with dementia during activities of daily living (Dizazzo-Miller et al., 2014, 2017) and providing home-based occupational therapy services using the person–environment framework (Dooley & Hinojosa, 2004).

Summary and Implications: The TAP is clinically useful for people with dementia and their caregivers as the intervention reduced behaviors that can lead to nursing home placement. However, recent meta-analyses including the TAP indicate that there is insufficient evidence to support the effectiveness of home-based therapy in improving quality of life among people with dementia (Bennett et al., 2019). Thus, there is a need to replicate studies involving the TAP or similar programs to further strengthen the evidence for community-based tailored occupational therapy interventions for people with dementia.

CLINICAL CASE: DISCHARGE PLANNING FOR AN AGING ADULT WITH DEMENTIA AND STROKE

Case History

Mr. John (he/him) is a 74-year-old Asian male diagnosed with vascular dementia and a history of hemorrhagic stroke affecting his right thalamus and parietal lobe about 10 years ago. He is now hospitalized for an acute urinary tract infection following recent episodes of delirium at home. He lives at home with his wife, whose health is also declining. Although he can ambulate and complete all of his activities of daily living, he has a high fall risk. He also has difficulty with transfers and learning new information and experiences pathological perceptions of pain on the left side of his body that make him irritable. How can the occupational therapist (OT) help this family prepare for future declines and train them to manage the progressive nature of this disorder?

Suggested Answer

The OT should facilitate a family-centered discussion of the pros and cons of discharge to home with in-home supports or to a subacute rehabilitation facility to reduce fall risk. Short-term intervention planning can be guided using the 4-month TAP. The first two sessions can focus on home evaluation and identification of other informal caregivers (adult children, grandchildren, or friends) to assist his wife daily at home. With an understanding of the environmental and social barriers affecting his physical safety and emotional well-being, the OT should develop activity prescriptions that can ameliorate deficits experienced from cognitive declines and reduce behavioral challenges. A component of that activity prescription could include the graded steps involved in sorting clean laundry with a grandchild once a week for 20 minutes. The TAP can reduce his wife's caregiving burden at home and potentially improve the quality of life of this aging family by reducing the risk for nursing home placement.

References

Bennett, S., Laver, K., Voigt-Radloff, S., Letts, L., Clemson, L., Graff, M., Wiseman, J., & Gitlin, L. (2019). Occupational therapy for people with dementia and their family carers provided at home: A systematic review and meta-analysis. *BMJ Open, 9*(11), Article e026308.

DiZazzo-Miller, R., Samuel, P. S., Barnas, J. M., & Welker, K. M. (2014). Addressing everyday challenges: Feasibility of a family caregiver training program for people with dementia. *American Journal of Occupational Therapy, 68*(2), 212–220.

DiZazzo-Miller, R., Winston, K., Winkler, S. L., & Donovan, M. L. (2017). Family caregiver training program (FCTP): A randomized controlled trial. *American Journal of Occupational Therapy, 71*(5), 7105190010p1–7105190010p10.

Dooley, N. R., & Hinojosa, J. (2004). Improving quality of life for persons with Alzheimer's disease and their family caregivers: Brief occupational therapy intervention. *American Journal of Occupational Therapy, 58*(5), 561–569.

Döpp, C. M., Graff, M. J., Teerenstra, S., Olde Rikkert, M. G., Nijhuis-van der Sanden, M. W., & Vernooij-Dassen, M. J. (2015). Effectiveness of a training package for implementing a community-based occupational therapy program in dementia: A cluster randomized controlled trial. *Clinical Rehabilitation, 29*(10), 974–986.

Gitlin, L. N., Arthur, P., Piersol, C., Hessels, V., Wu, S. S., Dai, Y., & Mann, W. C. (2018). Targeting behavioral symptoms and functional decline in dementia: A randomized clinical trial. *Journal of the American Geriatrics Society, 66*(2), 339–345. https://pubmed.ncbi.nlm.nih.gov/29192967/

Gitlin, L. N., Hodgson, N., Jutkowitz, E., & Pizzi, L. (2010). The cost-effectiveness of a nonpharmacologic intervention for individuals with dementia and family caregivers: The tailored activity program. *The American Journal of Geriatric Psychiatry, 18*(6), 510–519.

Gitlin, L. N., Mann, W. C., Vogel, W. B., & Arthur, P. B. (2013). A non-pharmacologic approach to address challenging behaviors of veterans with dementia: Description of the tailored activity program-VA randomized trial. *BMC Geriatrics, 13*(1), Article 96. https://pubmed.ncbi.nlm.nih.gov/24060106/

Gitlin, L. N., Winter, L., Dennis, M. P., Hodgson, N., & Hauck, W. W. (2010). A biobehavioral home-based intervention and the well-being of patients with dementia and their caregivers: The COPE randomized trial. *JAMA, 304*(9), 983–991.

Graff, M. J., Adang, E. M., Vernooij-Dassen, M. J., Dekker, J., Jönsson, L., Thijssen, M., Hoefnagels, W. H. L., & Olde Rikkert, M. G. (2008). Community occupational therapy for older patients with dementia and their care givers: Cost effectiveness study. *BMJ, 336*(7636), 134–138.

Graff, M. J., Vernooij-Dassen, M. J., Thijssen, M., Dekker, J., Hoefnagels, W. H., & Olde Rikkert, M. G. (2006). Community based occupational therapy for patients with dementia and their care givers: Randomised controlled trial. *BMJ, 333*(7580), 1196.

Novelli, M. M., Machado, S. C., Lima, G. B., Cantatore, L., Sena, B. P., Rodrigues, R. S., Rodrigues, C. I. B., Canon, M. B. F., Piersol, C. V., Nitrini, R., Yassuda, M. S., & Gitlin, L. N. (2018). Effects of the tailored activity program in Brazil (TAP-BR) for persons with dementia. *Alzheimer Disease & Associated Disorders, 32*(4), 339–345.

O'Connor, C. M., Clemson, L., Brodaty, H., Jeon, Y. H., Mioshi, E., & Gitlin, L. N. (2014). Use of the tailored activities program to reduce neuropsychiatric behaviors in dementia: An Australian protocol for a randomized trial to evaluate its effectiveness. *International Psychogeriatrics, 26*(5), 857–869.

9

Occupational Therapy for Patients with Parkinson's Disease

KAYOKO TAKAHASHI

The Occupational Therapy in Parkinson's Disease (OTiP) trial

The results of the present study suggest that occupational therapy improves self-perceived performance and satisfaction in daily activities, both immediately after the intervention (at 3 months) and after 6 months of follow-up in patients with Parkinson's disease.

STURKENBOOM, I. H., GRAFF, M. J., HENDRIKS, J. C., VEENHUIZEN, Y., MUNNEKE, M., BLOEM, B. R., & NIJHUIS-VAN DER SANDEN, M. W.; FOR THE OTiP STUDY GROUP. (2014). Efficacy of occupational therapy for patients with Parkinson's disease: A randomised controlled trial. *The Lancet Neurology, 13*(6), 557–566.

Original Paper: http://dx.doi.org/10.1016/S1474-4422(14)70055-9

Research Question: Is occupational therapy effective in improving perceived performance in daily activities of patients with Parkinson's disease?

Funding: Prinses Beatrix Spierfonds and Parkinson Vereniging.

Year Study Began: 2011

Year Study Published: 2014

Study Location: the Netherlands

Who Was Studied: Community-living patients with Parkinson's disease who report difficulty with daily activities. Patients' primary informal caregivers participated as available.

Who Was Excluded: Patients with the following characteristics were excluded:

- Diagnosis of atypical parkinsonism
- Received occupational therapy in the past 3 months
- Predominant disabling comorbidity
- Insufficient understanding of Dutch
- <24 Mini-Mental State Examination score

How Many Patients: 191

Study Overview: Patients were randomly assigned (2:1) to the intervention or control group (Figure 9.1).

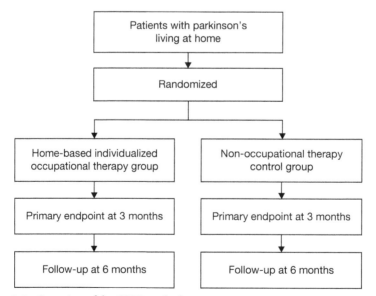

Figure 9.1. Overview of the OTiP study design.

Study Intervention: Individuals in the intervention received 10 weeks of home-based occupational therapy that followed the Dutch guidelines of occupational therapy for Parkinson's disease. In week 1, assessments were conducted, and the needs of both patients and caregivers were identified through interviews. In week 2, goal-setting and treatment-planning were done collaboratively by patients and therapists; and in weeks 3–10, the intervention was carried out. The intervention was focused on strategies for daily activity performance and adaptations of tasks, daily routines, or the environment (i.e., assistive devices). The content was individually tailored to patients, matching the nature of problems in prioritized activities, their coping style and capacity to change, as well as their environmental and social context. Individuals in the control condition received usual care with no occupational therapy.

Follow-Up: 3 months and 6 months

Endpoints:

Primary outcome:

- Self-perceived performance and satisfaction in daily activities, assessed with the Canadian Occupational Performance Measure (COPM; score 1 = poor performance and low satisfaction; 10 = very good performance and high satisfaction).

Secondary outcomes:

- Daily activity performance, measured with the Perceive, Recall, Plan, Perform System Phase 1.
- Participation in activities, measured with the Activity Card Sort and the Utrecht Scale for Evaluation of Rehabilitation-Participation Satisfaction Scale.
- Effect of fatigue, measured with the Fatigue Severity Scale.
- Proactive coping skills, measured with the Utrecht Proactive Coping Competence Scale.
- Mood, measured with the Beck Depression Inventory.
- Health-related quality of life, measured with the Parkinson's Disease Questionnaire 39 and the EuroQol: 5 Dimensions.
- Overall quality of life, measured with the Visual Analogue Scale.

RESULTS

- Self-perceived activity performance improved significantly over time within the intervention group (COPM performance score increased from 4.3 [interquartile range 3.5–5.0] at baseline to 5.8 [5.0–6.4] at 3 months and 5.7 [4.6–6.6] at 6 months) as opposed to the control group (COPM performance was 4.4 [3.8–5.0] at baseline, 4.6 [3.8–5.5] at 3 months, and 4.8 [4.0–5.5] at 6 months).
- Self-perceived activity satisfaction also improved significantly over time within the intervention group (COPM satisfaction score increased from 4.2 [interquartile range 3.2–4.8] at baseline to 5.6 [4.6–6.6] at 3 months and 5.7 [4.8–6.5] at 6 months) as opposed to the control group (COPM satisfaction was 4.3 [3.4–4.8] at baseline, 4.6 [3.8–5.8] at 3 months, and 4.8 [4.0–5.5] at 6 months).
- Differences between groups on self-perceived performance and satisfaction in daily activities (COPM) are shown in Table 9.1.
- There were no significant benefits in favor of the intervention for daily activity performance, participation in activities, fatigue, proactive coping skills, and mood (all, $p > 0.05$).
- Health-related quality of life (Parkinson's Disease Questionnaire-39) did not differ between groups, but the intervention group improved more than the control group at 6-month follow-up ($p = 0.056$).

Table 9.1. BETWEEN-GROUP COMPARISON ON SELF-PERCEIVED PERFORMANCE AND SATISFACTION IN DAILY ACTIVITIES

	Between-Group Difference at 3 Months		Between-Group Difference at 6 Months	
	Mean (95% CI)	p	Mean (95% CI)	p
COPM Performance scale	1.2 (0.8–1.6)	<0.0001	0.9 (0.5–1.3)	<0.0001
COPM Satisfaction scale	1.1 (0.7–1.5)	<0.0001	0.9 (0.5–1.3)	<0.0001

CI = confidence interval.

Criticisms and Limitations: Placebo effects may have contributed to the measured benefits of the intervention group since the control group was not offered an intervention. Recruitment procedures did not reflect clinical referral practices; thus, selection bias may have resulted. Study findings may lack generalizability to other countries as the research was conducted in the Netherlands.

Other Relevant Studies and Information:

- Meta-analyses have shown that occupational therapy interventions significantly improve activities of daily living and quality of life in patients with Parkinson's disease (Murphy & Tickle-Degnen, 2001; Tofani et al., 2020)
- A systematic review showed that quality of life can be improved through individualized, cognitive-behavioral interventions that target participant wellness initiatives and personal control (Foster et al., 2014). Likewise, a self-management program for people with Parkinson's disease improved health-related quality of life (Tickle-Degnen et al., 2010).
- Home-based occupational therapy consisting of client education using the Person–Environment–Occupation model resulted in improved endurance and body function, energy for work and leisure, and restoration of occupational roles in persons with Parkinson's disease. This result follows the patterns of task-specific response where patients improve on the exact task for which they were trained (Lowenstein & Tickle-Degnen, 2008).
- Self-management intervention for persons with Parkinson's disease should be individualized to match client needs and context such as health resources utilization, activities in home and community, and social support relationships (Tickle-Degnen et al., 2020).

Summary and Implications: This randomized controlled trial demonstrated that home-based individualized occupational therapy improves performance in and satisfaction with meaningful daily activities. These effects endure long term, 6 months after intervention conclusion. For people with Parkinson's disease, collaborative goal-setting and planning that aligns with the needs of both patients and caregivers and facilitation of self-management to improve task performance are key to long-term intervention effects.

CLINICAL CASE: SELF-MANAGEMENT STRATEGIES FOR PARKINSON'S DISEASE PATIENTS

Case History

Ms. Tanaka (she/her) is a 64-year-old woman diagnosed with Parkinson's disease who is attending outpatient occupational therapy. She enjoys household chores (especially cooking) and wants to resume these activities, but she states she is accustomed to the way she carried out her routines prior to Parkinson's disease and is not ready to change. Her upper limb endurance, trunk stability, and righting reflexes are reduced, resulting in poor balance in standing and sitting positions. In addition, as her disease has progressed, her function has declined. The patient states she cannot imagine how she could continue to cook, expressing anxiety and low confidence. As the occupational therapist, how should this patient be treated based on findings from this study?

Suggested Answer

This patient could benefit from learning compensatory methods to perform the activities she considers meaningful, such as cooking. This study suggests that strategy training in activities and adaptations to tasks or the environment could improve self-perceived performance and satisfaction in daily activities. The task-specific training should be individually tailored to suit this patient's limited readiness to change. While performing her meaningful activity (i.e., cooking), the occupational therapist should discuss with her how to problem-solve difficulties she is experiencing and offer strategies Ms. Tanaka would be willing to incorporate in her household chores routine. To address the environment, the occupational therapist could suggest use of a chair with armrests so that she can cook with added stability while sitting. Given her reluctance to make changes, practicing using a chair during occupational therapy sessions will provide her with direct experience that will facilitate incorporation of this strategy into her cooking routine. As this study showed long-term effects, Ms. Tanaka will likely be able to continue performing her meaningful activities after intervention.

References

Foster, E. R., Bedekar, M., & Tickle-Degnen, L. (2014). Systematic review of the effectiveness of occupational therapy–related interventions for people with Parkinson's disease. *American Journal of Occupational Therapy*, 68(1), 39–49. https://doi.org/10.5014/ajot.2014.008706

Lowenstein, N., & Tickle-Degnen, L. (2008). An occupational therapy home program for patients with Parkinson's disease. In M. Trail, E. Protas, & E. Lai (Eds.), Neurorehabilitation in Parkinson's disease: An evidence based treatment model (pp. 231–243). Slack.

Murphy, S., & Tickle-Degnen, L. (2001). The effectiveness of occupational therapy–related treatments for persons with Parkinson's disease: A meta-analytic review. *American Journal of Occupational Therapy*, 55, 385–392.

Tickle-Degnen, L., Ellis, T., Saint-Hilaire, M. H., Thomas, C. A., & Wagenaar, R. C. (2010). Self-management rehabilitation and health-related quality of life in Parkinson's disease: A randomized controlled trial. *Movement Disorders*, 25(2), 194–204. https://doi.org/10.1002/mds.22940

Tickle-Degnen, L., Stevenson, M. T., Gunnery, S. D., Saint-Hilaire, M., Thomas, C. A., Sprague Martinez, L., Habermann, B., & Naumova, E. N. (2020). Profile of social self-management practices in daily life with Parkinson's disease is associated with symptom severity and health quality of life. *Disability and Rehabilitation, 43*(22), 3212–3224. https://doi.org/10.1080/09638288.2020.1741035

Tofani, M., Ranieri, A., Fabbrini, G., Berardi, A., Pelosin, E., Valente, D., Fabbrini, A., Costanzo, M., & Galeoto, G. (2020). Efficacy of occupational therapy interventions on quality of life in patients with Parkinson's disease: A systematic review and meta-analysis. *Movement Disorders: Clinical Practice, 7*(8), 891–901. https://doi.org/10.1002/mdc3.13089

SECTION 2

Health and Wellness

Chronic physical and mental health conditions are the leading cause of disability and mortality in the United States, and lifestyle risk factors such as diet, physical activity, sleep, and substance use play a significant role in the development and progression of these conditions (Ford et al., 2013). In response to this trend, health and wellness has been identified by the American Occupational Therapy Association (AOTA) as an "area of practice primed for further development" (AOTA, 2020) encompassing a broad swath of occupational therapy (OT) interventions. These include preventing functional declines among older adults, preventing and managing chronic conditions to reduce the likelihood that they will cause disabling complications, and facilitating wellness among those challenged by occupational imbalances inherent in much of modern society.

While the potential for OT to contribute to health and wellness is significant, it is perhaps the least-developed practice area within OT, with an evidence base still in its infancy. The five papers selected for inclusion in this section span a wide range of study designs, intervention approaches, and populations. Among them, a few common themes are noted.

Chronic conditions are an overall focus, with research on diabetes, arthritis, multimorbidity, and a scoping review inclusive of multiple chronic conditions such as arthritis, chronic obstructive pulmonary disease, depression, and heart failure. Research on OT interventions for individuals, groups, and populations without a particular medical condition is still underdeveloped, with the important exception of the Well Elderly Study (as discussed below).

As the evidence base is still relatively new, studies generally lacked the degree of rigor present in more established areas of OT research. One exception was in the area of arthritis care (both autoimmune and degenerative), which has a robust evidence base with multiple large-scale randomized controlled trials; the Hammond & Freeman article is a strong exemplar of this body of research. Beyond arthritis, aside from one randomized controlled trial in diabetes included in this book (Pyatak et al.), most research in this practice area has been methodologically less rigorous, limited predominantly to case studies, small-scale pilot and feasibility studies, and quasi-experimental clinical outcomes research.

A number of influential papers within the realm of health and wellness were not included in this text because of our focus on peer-reviewed original research articles. These include position statements (e.g., Halle, 2020), theoretical papers (e.g., Mackenzie et al., 2013), and editorials (e.g., Hildenbrand & Lamb, 2013). While critical to advancing the role of OT in settings supporting health and wellness, such as population health, prevention, and primary healthcare, these papers were outside the scope of our mission in *50 Studies*, which (as its title suggests) is focused on empirical research.

Our team faced a decision about a groundbreaking work bridging the Productive Aging and Health and Wellness sections of this book, Clark et al.'s article reporting on the Well Elderly Study. We ultimately decided that while the Well Elderly Study was crucial to understanding the evidence base in productive aging, it should surely also be considered the seminal modern work representing OT's potential to contribute to wellness and prevention.

Finally, some newer works relevant to OT practice in health and wellness were considered for inclusion in this section, most notably a burgeoning international literature advancing OT practice in primary care settings (e.g., Bolt et al., 2019; Lindström & Bernhardsson, 2018). While a foundational study in primary care by Donnelly et al. was selected for inclusion in this book, we felt that the impact of these more recent works is, as of yet, unclear. Given recent trends in healthcare emphasizing prevention and chronic care, we anticipate that the evidence base in this area will continue to expand, demonstrating OT's important contributions to this area of practice.

References

American Occupational Therapy Association (2020). Occupational therapy in the promotion of health and well-being. *American Journal of Occupational Therapy, 74*(3), 7403420010p1–7403420010p14. doi: https://doi.org/10.5014/ajot.2020.743003

Bolt, M., Ikking, T., Baaijen, R., & Saenger, S. (2019). Scoping review: Occupational therapy interventions in primary care. *Primary Health Care Research & Development, 20*, Article e28. https://doi.org/10.1017/S146342361800049X

Ford, E. S., Croft, J. B., Posner, S. F., Goodman, R. A., & Giles, W. H. (2013). Co-occurrence of leading lifestyle-related chronic conditions among adults in the United States, 2002–2009. *Preventing Chronic Disease, 10*, Article E60. https://doi.org/10.5888/pcd10.120316

Halle, A. (2020). Role of occupational therapy in primary care. *American Journal of Occupational Therapy, 74*(Supplement_3), Article 7413410040. https://doi.org/10.5014/ajot.2020.74S3001

Hildenbrand, W. C., & Lamb, A. J. (2013). Occupational therapy in prevention and wellness: Retaining relevance in a new health care world. *American Journal of Occupational Therapy, 67*(3), 266–271. https://doi.org/10.5014/ajot.2013.673001

Lindström, A. C., & Bernhardsson, S. (2018). Evidence-based practice in primary care occupational therapy: A cross-sectional survey in Sweden. *Occupational Therapy International, 2018*, Article 5376764. https://doi.org/10.1155/2018/5376764

Mackenzie, L., Clemson, L., & Roberts, C. (2013). Occupational therapists partnering with general practitioners to prevent falls: Seizing opportunities in primary health care. *Australian Occupational Therapy Journal, 60*(1), 66–70.

10

Scoping Review of Occupational Therapy Interventions for Chronic Diseases

CAROL SIEBERT

Interventions involving occupational therapy can improve function in BADLs and IADLs in people with COPD, RA, or multiple conditions. Occupational therapy can improve work outcomes for adults with depression and may improve social functioning in people with RA and COPD.... Taken together, the evidence suggests that occupational therapy can improve occupational outcomes in people with a range of chronic diseases.
HAND, C., LAW, M., & MCCOLL, M. A. (2011). Occupational therapy interventions for chronic diseases: A scoping review. *American Journal of Occupational Therapy, 65*(4), 428–436.

Original Paper: https://doi.org/10.5014/ajot.2011.002071

Research Question: Are community occupational therapy (OT) interventions effective in improving occupational outcomes for adults with selected chronic conditions?

Funding:

- Canadian Institutes of Health Research Institute of Aging and Institute of Musculoskeletal Health and Arthritis
- Ontario Rehabilitation Research Advisory Network/Ontario Neurotrauma Foundation
- Ministry of Health and Long Term Care, Ontario, Canada

Year Study Began: The earliest trial with a reported start date began in 1984 and the most recent in 2004. Eleven studies did not report a start date.

Year Study Published: The results of the individual trials were published during the 1990s and the first decade of the 2000s. The review was published in 2011.

Study Location: The reviewed trials were conducted in Canada, Denmark, Italy, the Netherlands, the United Kingdom, and the United States.

Who Was Studied: This was a scoping review of randomized clinical trials including OT (alone or as part of multidisciplinary intervention) for individuals with cardiovascular disease, chronic obstructive pulmonary disease (COPD), depression, or rheumatoid arthritis (RA).

Which Trials Were Included? A total of 141 articles were identified using an exhaustive search strategy. Studies were included if they focused on community/ outpatient interventions, were randomized controlled trials published in English, involved adults with cardiovascular disease, COPD, depression, diabetes, RA, or osteoarthritis (OA), and reported on occupational outcomes. Studies focusing exclusively on splinting or on cerebrovascular disease were excluded. This resulted in 17 articles reporting on 16 studies included in the review. Table 10.1 lists the studies by lead author and study name (if any), country, chronic condition addressed, and start date, if reported. As there are several studies by the same author or co-authors, a co-author and publication year are also included to distinguish among studies.

Table 10.1. Studies by Country, Condition Addressed, and Start Date

Lead Author	Country	Condition Addressed	Year Started
Austin	United Kingdom	Heart failure	Not reported
Bendstrup	Denmark	COPD	Not reported
De Buck	the Netherlands	RA	1999
Finnerty	United Kingdom	COPD	Not reported
Gitlin	United States	Multiple	2000
Griffiths	United Kingdom	COPD	Not reported
Hammond & Freeman (2001, 2004)	United Kingdom	RA	Not reported
Hammond (2004)	United Kingdom	RA	Not reported
Hammond (1999)	United Kingdom	RA	Not reported
Hammond (2002)	United Kingdom	RA	Not reported
Helewa	Canada	RA	1984
Kraaimaat	the Netherlands	RA	Not reported

Lead Author	Country	Condition Addressed	Year Started
Li (2005)	Canada	RA	1999
Li (2006)	Canada	RA	Not reported
Masiero	Italy	RA	2004
Schene	the Netherlands	Depression	Not reported

Study Intervention: In each study, the intervention group received either OT alone or as part of a multidisciplinary intervention, while the control group received usual care. The multidisciplinary interventions included as few as one or as many as five other professionals. The studies focused on COPD (three studies), depression (one study), heart failure, and RA (ten studies). One study focused on multiple conditions, including cardiovascular disease, OA, and diabetes. The interventions included OT delivered individually (two studies), OT delivered both individually and to a group (two studies), either OT or physical therapy delivered individually (two studies), OT delivered solely to a group (four studies), OT delivered individually as part of a multidisciplinary intervention (one study), and OT with other disciplines delivering the intervention to a group (five studies). Duration of intervention ranged from 2 weeks to 1 year.

RESULTS

- Six studies, all addressing RA, had non-significant results.
- Ten studies had at least one significant result. These studies addressed heart failure, RA, COPD, depression, and multiple chronic conditions.
- In general, significant improvements were noted in two areas of function: activities of daily living (ADL)/instrumental ADL (IADL) performance and social participation (Table 10.2).

Table 10.2. RESULTS BY OUTCOME DOMAIN AND STUDY

Outcome Domain	Study	Disease Focus	Significant Improvement	Insignificant Improvement
ADL/IADL	Bendstrup	COPD	x	
	Hammond & Freeman (2001, 2004)	RA	x	
	Gitlin, Project ABLE	Multiple	x	
	Helewa	RA	x	

Outcome Domain	Study	Disease Focus	Significant Improvement	Insignificant Improvement
Work	Schene	Depression	x	
	de Buck	RA		x
	Hammond (2004)	RA		x
	Masiero	RA		x
Social Function	Griffiths	COPD	x	
	Masiero	RA	x	
Physical Function or Physical Health	Griffiths	COPD	x	
	Masiero	RA	x	
	Hammond & Freeman, (2001, 2004)	RA		x
	Hammond (2002)	RA		x
	Hammond (1999)	RA		x
	Hammond (2004)	RA		x
	Helewa	RA		x
	Li (2005, 2006)	RA		x
	de Buck	RA		x
	Gitlin	Multiple		x
Psychological Health	de Buck	RA	x	
	Griffiths	COPD	x	
Health Status or Quality of Life	Austin	Heart failure	x	
	Finnerty	COPD	x	
	Griffiths	COPD	x	
	Bendstrup	COPD		x
	Kraaimaat	RA		x
	Li (2005)	RA		x

Criticisms and Limitations:

- Diversity of outcome domains and measures limits generalization of results or comparison among studies.
- Four studies were very small: $n < 40$, with fewer than 20 participants in each group.

- Multidisciplinary group interventions did not consistently specify the role or contribution of OT; thus, it is unclear whether/how the observed outcomes may be attributed to OT.
- Some studies used study-specific outcome measures rather than standardized or widely recognized measures.
- Two studies used occupational therapists and physical therapists interchangeably to deliver intervention, so not all intervention participants received OT.

Other Relevant Studies and Information:

- In working-age adults with RA, individual OT for six to eight sessions led to significantly greater improvement in occupational outcomes and work outcomes compared to usual care. The intervention group also saw significant improvement in multiple arthritis pain and impact measures and in quality of life at follow-up as compared to baseline (Macedo et al., 2009).
- Among ethnically diverse, low–socioeconomic status young adults with diabetes, individual OT over 6 months resulted in significant improvements in blood glucose control, diabetes quality of life, and habit strength of checking blood glucose over usual care (Pyatak et al., 2018).
- A study of older African Americans with mild cognitive impairment, low medication adherence, and poor blood glucose control evaluated individual OT for 6 months compared to diabetes self-management education (DSME; control group). The study found equivalence of OT behavioral intervention and DSME, with 61% of OT participants and 48% of control participants having a clinically significant reduction in blood glucose (Rovner et al., 2020).
- The CAPABLE trial evaluated a multidisciplinary intervention among older adults with multiple ADL/IADL limitations. Participants received individual home visits from OT (up to six visits) and a registered nurse (four visits) with handy person services for repairs and home modifications as identified by OT over 6 months. The intervention group improved on all outcomes: ADL, IADL, falls efficacy, and quality of life (Szanton et al., 2011).

Summary and Implications: This scoping review identified 16 studies involving OT interventions addressing high-prevalence/disabling chronic conditions. The diversity of study designs and outcome measures makes it difficult to generalize results. Common characteristics of the interventions include a focus on coping with activities and tailoring of interventions to individual participants. Taken together, the studies suggest that OT may contribute to improved ADL/IADL, social and psychological function, and quality of life for adults living with chronic conditions. More studies of OT interventions for chronic conditions are needed with a clearly defined methodology, robust sample size, and use of widely recognized outcome measures.

CLINICAL CASE: COMMUNITY PROGRAM TO MANAGE DAILY DEMANDS

Case History

Rasika (she/her), a 63-year-old woman with COPD and depression, works as an administrator on a college campus. She is considering having to retire early as she is having increasing difficulty managing daily activities. She reports "no energy" and has been overusing her inhaled medications, telling her doctor that "I just can't catch my breath." Her healthcare provider suggests that she participate in a program involving nursing, psychology, and OT, including both group and individual sessions with each discipline. Based on the results of the scoping review of OT interventions for chronic diseases, what can you tell Rasika about the possible risks and benefits of participating in the program?

Suggested Answer

The scoping review suggests that such interventions that include OT may produce modest improvement in performance of daily activities, psychological health, and quality of life. Such programs focus on coping with daily activities. They also provide social support. Interventions are tailored to the participant. They may include follow-up contacts by phone or visits to encourage application of the program content to daily life. There is no guarantee that she will benefit from such a program or that any benefit or improvement will be sustained, but the program may help her develop more effective strategies to manage her condition and with daily activities, whether she continues to work or decides to retire.

References

Austin, J., Williams, R., Ross, L., Moseley, L., & Hutchison, S. (2005). Randomised controlled trial of cardiac rehabilitation in elderly patients with heart failure. *European Journal of Heart Failure, 7*(3), 411–417.

Bendstrup, K. E., Ingemann Jensen, J., Holm, S., & Bengtsson, B. (1997). Out-patient rehabilitation improves activities of daily living, quality of life and exercise tolerance in chronic obstructive pulmonary disease. *European Respiratory Journal, 10*, 2801–2806.

de Buck, P. D., le Cessie, S., van den Hout, W., Peeters, A., Ronday, H., Westedt, M., Breedveld, F. C., & Vliet Vlieland, T. P. M. (2005). Randomized comparison of a multidisciplinary job retention vocational rehabilitation program with usual outpatient care in patients with chronic arthritis at risk for job loss. *Arthritis Care and Research, 53*, 682–690. https://doi.org/10.1002/art.21452

Finnerty, J. P., Keeping, I., Bullough, I., & Jones, J. (2001). The effectiveness of outpatient pulmonary rehabilitation in chronic lung disease: A randomized controlled trial. *Chest, 119*, 1705–1710. https://doi.org/10.1378/chest.119.6.1705

Gitlin, L. N., Winter, L., Dennis, M. P., Corcoran, M., Schinfeld, S., & Hauck, W. W. (2006). A randomized trial of a multicomponent home intervention to reduce functional difficulties in older adults. *Journal of the American Geriatrics Society, 54*, 809–816. https://doi.org/10.1111/j.1532-5415.2006.00703.x

Griffiths, T. L., Burr, M. L., Campbell, I. A., Lewis Jenkins, V., Mullins, J., Shiels, K., Turner-Lawlor, P. J., Payne, N., Newcombe, R. G., Lonescu, A. A., Thomas, J., & Tunbridge, J. (2000). Results at 1 year of outpatient multidisciplinary pulmonary rehabilitation: A randomised controlled trial. *Lancet, 355*, 362–368. https://doi.org/10.1016/S0140-6736(99)07042-7

Hammond, A., & Freeman, K. (2001). One-year outcomes of a randomized controlled trial of an educational–behavioural joint protection programme for people with rheumatoid arthritis. *Rheumatology, 40*, 1044–1051. https://doi.org/10.1093/rheumatology/40.9.1044

Hammond, A., & Freeman, K. (2004). The long-term outcomes from a randomized controlled trial of an educational–behavioural joint protection programme for people with rheumatoid arthritis. *Clinical Rehabilitation, 18*, 520–528. https://doi.org/10.1191/0269215504cr766oa

Hammond, A., Jeffreson, P., Jones, N., Gallagher, J., & Jones, T. (2002). Clinical applicability of an educational–behavioural joint protection programme for people with rheumatoid arthritis. *British Journal of Occupational Therapy, 65*, 405–412.

Hammond, A., Lincoln, N., & Sutcliffe, L. (1999). A crossover trial evaluating an educational–behavioural joint protection programme for people with rheumatoid arthritis. *Patient Education and Counseling, 37*, 19–32. https://doi.org/10.1016/S0738-3991(98)00093-7

Hammond, A., Young, A., & Kidao, R. (2004). A randomized controlled trial of occupational therapy for people with early rheumatoid arthritis. *Annals of the Rheumatic Diseases, 63*, 23–30. https://doi.org/10.1136/ard.2002.001511

Helewa, A., Goldsmith, C. H., Tugwell, P., Hanes, B., Bombardier, C., Smythe, H. A., & Lee, P. (1991). Effects of occupational therapy home service on patients with rheumatoid arthritis. *Lancet, 337*, 1453–1456. https://doi.org/10.1016/0140-6736(91)93138-Y

Kraaimaat, F. W., Brons, M. R., Geenen, R., & Bijlsma, J. W. (1995). The effect of cognitive behavior therapy in patients with rheumatoid arthritis. *Behaviour Research and Therapy, 33*, 487–495. https://doi.org/10.1016/0005-7967(94)00094-Z

Li, L. C., Davis, A. M., Lineker, S., Coyte, P. C., & Bombardier, C. (2005). Outcomes of home-based rehabilitation provided by primary therapists for patients with rheumatoid arthritis: Pilot study. *Physiotherapy Canada, 57,* 255–264. https://doi.org/10.3138/ptc.57.4.255

Li, L. C., Davis, A. M., Lineker, S. C., Coyte, P. C., & Bombardier, C. (2006). Effectiveness of the primary therapist model for rheumatoid arthritis rehabilitation: A randomized controlled trial. *Arthritis and Rheumatism, 56,* 42–52. https://doi.org/10.1002/art.21692

Macedo, A. M., Oakley, S. P., Panayi, G. S., & Kirkham, B. W. (2009). Functional and work outcomes improve in patients with rheumatoid arthritis who receive targeted, comprehensive occupational therapy. *Arthritis & Rheumatism, 61*(11), 1522–1530. https://doi.org/10.1002/art.24563

Masiero, S., Boniolo, A., Wassermann, L., Machiedo, H., Volante, D., & Punzi, L. (2007). Effects of an educational–behavioral joint protection program on people with moderate to severe rheumatoid arthritis: A randomized controlled trial. *Clinical Rheumatology, 26,* 2043–2050. https://doi.org/10.1007/s10067-007-0615-0

Pyatak, E. A., Carandang, K., Vigen, C. L., Blanchard, J., Díaz, J., Concha-Chavez, A., Sequeira, P. A., Wood, J. R., Whittemore, R., Spruijt-Metz, D., & Peters, A. L. (2018). Occupational therapy intervention improves glycemic control and quality of life among young adults with diabetes: The Resilient, Empowered, Active Living with Diabetes (REAL Diabetes) randomized controlled trial. *Diabetes Care, 41*(4), 696–704. https://doi.org/10.2337/dc17-1634

Rovner, B. W., Casten, R. J., Piersol, C. V., White, N., Kelley, M., & Leiby, B. E. (2020). Improving glycemic control in African Americans with diabetes and mild cognitive impairment. *Journal American Geriatrics Society, 68,* 1015–1022. https://doi.org/10.1111/jgs.16339

Schene, A. H., Koeter, M. W. J., Kikkert, M. J., Swinkels, J. A., & McCrone, P. (2007). Adjuvant occupational therapy for work-related major depression works: Randomized trial including economic evaluation. *Psychological Medicine, 37,* 351–362. https://doi.org/10.1017/S0033291706009366

Szanton, S. L., Thorpe, R. J., Boyd, C., Tanner, E. K., Leff, B. Agree, E., Qian-Li, X., Allen, J. K., Selaki, C. L., Weiss, C. O., Guralnik, J. M., & Gitlin, L. N. (2011). Community aging in place, advancing better living for elders: A bio-behavioral-environmental intervention to improve function and health-related quality of life in disabled older adults. *Journal of the American Geriatrics Society, 59,* 2314–2320. https://doi.org/10.1111/j.1532-5415.2011.03698.x

11

The Integration of Occupational Therapy into Primary Care

ELIZABETH A. PYATAK AND DANIEL PADILLA VEGA

Processes that were seen to support the integration of occupational therapy included co-location, a common EMR, formal and informal communication structures and team meetings. Each of these processes naturally facilitated the integration of occupational therapy into the team by building trust, understanding and familiarity.

DONNELLY, C., BRENCHLEY, C., CRAWFORD, C., & LETTS, L. (2013). The integration of occupational therapy into primary care: A multiple case study design. *BMC Family Practice, 14*(1), Article 60.

Original Paper: https://doi.org/10.1186/1471-2296-14-60

Research Question: What structures and processes support the integration of occupational therapy (OT) in family health teams (FHTs; an innovative model of interprofessional primary care)?

Funding: The Primary Healthcare Seed Funding

Year Study Began: 2012

Year Study Published: 2013

Study Location: Ontario, Canada

Who Was Studied: Members of four FHTs (interprofessional primary care health teams). Disciplines of the FHT members included:

- Occupational therapists
- Executive directors
- Lead physicians
- Other members of the FHTs who provided collaborative patient care (i.e., nurse practitioner, social worker, dietician, diabetes educator)

Who Was Excluded: FHTs not employing occupational therapists were excluded.

How Many Participants: 20

Study Overview: Four FHTs were identified to study the role and integration of OT on FHTs. Cases were purposefully sampled to ensure diversity of setting types, location, number of patients, number of sites, referral process, co-location, occupational therapist's clinical experience, and electronic medical record (EMR) access. All occupational therapists working at their respective FHT participated and acted as the main liaison and coordinator for the study. Any team member who collaborated with the occupational therapist was asked to participate. Data collection included semi-structured interviews, document analyses, questionnaires, and an FHT profile. Within-case and cross-case analyses were conducted to identify patterns and code data to understand how occupational therapists are integrated into primary care and structures to support the integration (Table 11.1).

Table 11.1. DESCRIPTION OF CASE STUDY SITES

Family Health Team	Case 1	Case 2	Case 3	Case 4
Setting	Very large rural community	Small urban community	Large rural community	Urban academic
Number of sites	22	4	4	2
Patients	46,000	7,200	26,500	28,000
OT clinical experience	>15 years	<5 years	<5 years	>20 years
EMR integration	Yes	Yes (3 of 4 sites)	No	Yes
Co-location	Physicians: No Other health team members: Yes	Physicians: No Other health team members: Yes	Physicians: No Other health team members: Yes	Physicians: Yes Other health team members: Yes

Family Health Team	Case 1	Case 2	Case 3	Case 4
Referrals to OT	Physician, other health providers via EMR and administered through central office	Any team member or patient self-referral directly via EMR	Physician, other health providers via fax through central administration	Any team member or patient self-referral directly via EMR

Study Intervention: Not applicable.

Follow-Up: Data were collected over a 4-month period from February to May 2012.

Endpoints: The primary outcomes of interest were the structures and processes that supported integration of OT onto FHTs.

Understanding Occupational Therapy

- An understanding of the role of OT and the services available for patients resulted in increased referrals, utilization of services, level of respect, and integration into the team.
- Occupational therapists provided education to the team about OT via presentations, educational rounds, meet and greets, brochures, information letters, and information booths.
- Understanding of OT was enhanced in settings that offered research and teaching opportunities through resident training, interprofessional teaching rounds, education clinics, and student mentorship.
- Identifying physician champions was critical for integration of OT as physicians were key sources of referrals and often viewed by the team to have greater authority and credibility.

A Culture of Collaboration

- Purposeful interprofessional collaboration and support was vital for the integration of OT into FHTs.
- Aligning OT services with current on-site programs (i.e., health promotion, prevention programs, chronic disease management, etc.) provided opportunities to collaborate with team members, develop

new programs, and connect with physicians involved in specific programs.

- Collaboration with OT colleagues within and outside the FHT via resources, consultations, and sharing strategies to support integration into the team provided professional support and confidence.

Communication and Trust

- An accessible EMR was critical for the integration of OT as it facilitated communication and collaboration with physicians and team members through messaging and patient records.
- The opportunity for team members to interact face to face through co-location, formal meetings, and social gatherings provided opportunities for team-building and enabled team members to build trust, understanding, and communication that helped integrate OT into the primary care team.

RESULTS

The study identified three primary themes that influenced the integration of occupational therapists on FHTs.

Criticisms and Limitations: The results of the study may not be broadly generalizable as its scope was small; a larger study may have produced additional insights regarding structures and processes supporting integration. Additionally, the study was conducted at one time point, when OT was initially integrated within FHTs. A longitudinal study would provide further understanding of interprofessional integration over time and its impact on health outcomes.

Other Relevant Studies and Information:

- Occupational therapists in FHTs function as "generalists" that provide one-on-one care while integrating themselves into and supporting development of existing programs and group interventions (Donnelly et al., 2014).
- OT in a primary care setting increases access to OT services that otherwise would not be readily available to community members (Donnelly et al., 2014).
- Outreach and educating healthcare providers about OT's role and scope of practice helped depict the unique skill set of OT in chronic disease management and increase referrals for services (Mirza et al., 2020).

- Co-location, EMR integration, and support from clinic leadership facilitated successful integration of OT within a safety-net primary care clinic, where patients with diabetes who received OT demonstrated improved blood glucose levels, diabetes self-care, and health status (Pyatak et al., 2019).

Summary and Implications: The integration of occupational therapists within primary care teams requires the development of trust, understanding, and communication. Occupational therapists entering primary care settings need to develop their role through educating physicians and other team members about the role of OT and services provided. Structures and processes including co-location, existing team-based patient programs, EMR integration, support from occupational therapist colleagues, formal and informal communication, and team meetings were found to support the integration of OT. This study contributes to the existing literature regarding the integration of OT in primary care as well as the structures and processes that support interprofessional collaboration within primary healthcare settings.

CLINICAL CASE: ESTABLISHING OT IN PRIMARY CARE

Case History

An occupational therapist with 1 year of clinical experience is offered a new position in primary care at an urban community clinic providing care to an underserved population. This is the first time the clinic team will include an occupational therapist. Many of the team members are unaware of the scope of practice of OT and what potential services the occupational therapist can offer to their patients. The clinic medical director has been an advocate for OT and wants to ensure a smooth integration into the team. Based on Donnelly et al.'s findings, how can the occupational therapist help to ensure a successful integration within the primary care team?

Suggested Answer

Before taking the position, the occupational therapist should inquire whether there are structures in place that will support his integration onto the team. Co-location with physicians and other clinic team members and full EMR access are two important structures that will facilitate his success as a new team member. Since he will be the only occupational therapist at the clinic, he should also consider whether he has OT colleagues working in primary care who can provide support and mentorship as he establish his role on the primary care team. Finally, after taking the position, the occupational therapist should identify existing patient programs where he can provide added value; inform his team members about his role and scope of practice through formal and informal communications such as daily rounds, team meetings, and EMR messaging; and seek to develop trusting relationships with physicians and other team members.

References

Donnelly, C. A., Brenchley, C. L., Crawford, C. N., & Letts, L. J. (2014). The emerging role of occupational therapy in primary care. *Canadian Journal of Occupational Therapy/ Revue Canadienne d'Ergotherapie, 81*(1), 51–61. https://doi.org/10.1177/000841741 4520683

Mirza, M., Gecht-Silver, M., Keating, E., Krischer, A., Kim, H., & Kottorp, A. (2020). Feasibility and preliminary efficacy of an occupational therapy intervention for older adults with chronic conditions in a primary care clinic. *American Journal of Occupational Therapy, 74*(5), 7405205030p1–7405205030p13. https://doi.org/ 10.5014/ajot.2020.039842

Pyatak, E., King, M., Vigen, C. L. P., Salazar, E., Diaz, J., Schepens Niemiec, S. L., Blanchard, J., Jordan, M. K., Banerjee, J., & Shukla, J. (2019). Addressing diabetes in primary care: Hybrid effectiveness–implementation study of Lifestyle Redesign' occupational therapy. *American Journal of Occupational Therapy, 73*(5), 7305185020p1– 7305185020p12. https://doi.org/10.5014/ajot.2019.037317

12

An Occupational Therapy–Led Self-Management Program to Support People with Multiple Chronic Conditions (MCCs) in Primary Care

ELIZABETH A. PYATAK AND ELISSA S. LEE

The OPTIMAL Study

OPTIMAL significantly improved frequency of activity participation, self-efficacy and quality of life for patients with multimorbidity. Further work is required to test the sustainability of these effects over time but this study indicates that it is a promising intervention that can be delivered in primary care and community settings.

GARVEY, J., CONNOLLY, D., BOLAND, F., & SMITH, S. M. (2015). OPTIMAL, an occupational therapy led self-management support programme for people with multimorbidity in primary care: A randomized controlled trial. *BMC Family Practice, 16*(1), Article 59.

Original Paper: https://link.springer.com/article/10.1186/s12875-015-0267-0

Research Question: Can a community-based occupational therapy self-management support program help to address challenges of living among adults with?

Funding: This study was funded by the Health Research Board Research Training Fellowship for Healthcare Professionals and the Health Research Board Centre for Primary Care Research. The Health Research Board is the lead agency in Ireland supporting and funding health research.

Year Study Began: 2013

Year Study Published: 2015

Study Location: Participants were referred by primary care clinicians in three primary care network areas in Dublin, Ireland.

Who Was Studied: Sixty-three participants with MCCs were referred by primary care clinicians, with 50 enrolling in the study. Inclusion criteria included being over 18 years of age, having two or more chronic conditions, and receiving four or more repeat medications.

Who Was Excluded: Patients who were unable to travel to the center where groups were delivered were excluded.

How Many Patients: 50

Study Overview: See Figure 12.1.

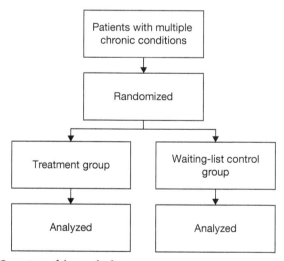

Figure 12.1. Overview of the study design.

Study Intervention: Participants randomized to the treatment group were provided with a weekly 3-hour program for 6 weeks held in local community health centers. Groups were professionally led, facilitated by community-based occupational therapists, and incorporated elements of peer support available through the group format.

Sessions focused on supporting self-management, which included discussion of areas identified as problematic for people with chronic conditions such as fatigue and energy management, communication with health professionals, anxiety, and medication management. The occupational therapists facilitated active group discussion to engage participants in examining how these areas impact activity performance and participation. Participants set weekly achievable and realistic goals during group sessions, and occupational therapists provided practical strategies on how to maintain participation in valued activities.

Participants allocated to the control group were placed on a waiting list and were invited to attend an OPTIMAL course when the trial was complete.

Follow-Up: Two weeks post-intervention

Endpoints:

- Primary outcome: frequency of activity participation
- Secondary outcomes: healthcare utilization, activity performance and satisfaction, mental health, chronic disease self-efficacy

---

RESULTS

- Of the 26 participants in the intervention group, 20 (77%) attended at least one session and 16 (62%) attended three or more sessions.
- The study found a significant increase in frequency of activity participation (Frenchay Activities Index; FAI) within the treatment group; in examining FAI subscales, the only significant difference was in domestic activity participation (e.g., household chores, meal preparation) (Table 12.1).
- For secondary outcomes, there were significant differences between intervention and control groups for activity performance and satisfaction (Canadian Occupational Performance Measure [COPM]), changes in instrumental activities of daily living (Nottingham Extended Activities of

Daily Living [NEADL]), chronic disease self-efficacy (Stanford Chronic Disease Self-Efficacy Scale [SSE]), and quality of life (EuroQol Visual Analogue Scale [EQ-VAS]).

- No significant difference was seen for anxiety and depression (Hospital Anxiety and Depression Scale [HADS]) or health-related quality of life (EuroQol–5 Dimensions [EQ-5D]), though results in the EQ-5D indicated a trend toward improvement.
- No significant differences were identified in healthcare utilization (both groups revealed high levels of service utilization, particularly in family practice services), though this could be attributed to the short follow-up time period and the fact that the study was not powered to detect differences in this outcome.
- The Goal Attainment Scale was only used among those who attended the intervention, with significant differences found between baseline and follow-up ($p \leq 0.01$). Of 20 participants, 19 had significant achievement in their identified goals, which averaged three per participant. Commonly cited goals included improving fitness levels, losing weight, increasing confidence levels, improving diet, and developing a more structured daily routine.

Table 12.1. A Comparison of FAI Baseline and Follow-Up Scores

	Intervention Group ($n = 22$)		Control Group ($n = 22$)		p
	Baseline	**Follow-up**	**Baseline**	**Follow-up**	
FAI total (0–45)[a]	21.3 (7.9)	24.9 (7.4)	19.8 (6.5)	18.9 (7.2)	<0.01
COPM Performance (1–10)[a]	4.1 (1.4)	5.8 (1.8)	4.4 (1.3)	4.1 (1.4)	0.02
COPM Satisfaction (1–10)[a]	3.2 (1.9)	5.6 (2.0)	3.1 (1.7)	3.4 (1.9)	0.02
NEADL (0–66)[a]	43.1 (12.4)	47.2 (11.9)	44.5 (10.8)	40.7 (10.7)	0.02
HADS (0–21)[b]	16.7 (8.3)	15.6 (8.3)	17.1 (6.9)	16.7 (8.2)	0.49
SSE (1–10)[a]	5.6 (1.9)	6.8 (1.5)	5.8 (2.0)	5.3 (1.9)	0.02
EQ-VAS (0–100)[a]	49.9 (22.9)	65.7 (20.2)	54.3 (20.8)	50.5 (16.3)	0.02

[a]Higher scores indicate better performance.
[b]Lower scores indicate better performance.

Criticisms and Limitations: The short referral period may have led to selection bias as clinicians may have been more likely to refer patients who were better known to them. The study had a short follow-up period, so it is not possible to ascertain whether benefits were sustained over time. Lastly, outcome assessors were not blinded, which may have led to bias.

Other Relevant Studies and Information:

- The OPTIMAL program's pilot study indicated similarly promising results in improving activity frequency, self-efficacy, and satisfaction and included the full details of course content (Toole et al., 2012).
- An occupational therapy program providing self-management support in primary care for individuals with diabetes (who also typically had MCCs) demonstrated improvements in blood glucose levels, blood pressure, overall health status, and health behaviors such as medication adherence and checking blood glucose (Pyatak et al., 2019).
- Though focused on a different population, a self-management program led by occupational therapists for patients post-stroke in the United States demonstrated significant short-term increases in health-related self-efficacy and participation self-efficacy (Wolf et al., 2016).

Summary and Implications: Among adults with MCCs referred from primary care, a community-based occupational therapy self-management support program led to improved activity participation, self-efficacy, and quality of life. For individuals with MCCs, maintaining engagement in daily activities (e.g., household chores and meal preparation) is essential to maintaining functional independence and quality of life.

CLINICAL CASE: PROMOTING HEALTH OF OLDER LIVING IN AN INDEPENDENT-LIVING COMMUNITY

Case History

An administrator at a large health system is interested in implementing a series of evidence-based interventions for patients with MCCs within primary care, to prevent further complications. Research shows that MCCs are an independent predictor of adverse outcomes, including poor quality of life, mortality, and disability. The health system sees a diverse range of patient populations, many of whom have poorly controlled diabetes, high cholesterol, and high blood pressure and are overweight/obese. The health system is participating in a pay-for-performance program that has selected comprehensive diabetes care (hemoglobin A1c), obesity (body mass index), and reported tobacco use as its performance measures. What sort of programming should the health system invest in to address this need?

Suggested Answer

This study, as well as others, would support integrating an occupational therapist into primary care settings to implement a professionally led prevention program similar to OPTIMAL for patients with MCCs. The administrator knows from the research that there are benefits to peer-led groups but that they could have adverse effects if participants perceive their peers having dissimilar lifestyles, which applies to this health system's patient population. Patients would be referred to the program by primary care clinicians. The occupational therapist would lead group sessions derived from the OPTIMAL program, with a focus on the patients' needs and interests as well as the performance measures.

References

Pyatak, E., King, M., Vigen, C. L., Salazar, E., Diaz, J., Schepens Niemiec, S. L., Blanchard, J., Jordan, M. K., Banerjee, J., & Shukla, J. (2019). Addressing diabetes in primary care: Hybrid effectiveness–implementation study of Lifestyle Redesign® occupational therapy. *American Journal of Occupational Therapy*, 73(5), 7305185020p1–7305185020p12. https://doi.org/10.5014/ajot.2019.037317

Toole, L. O., Connolly, D., & Smith, S. (2012). Impact of an occupation-based self-management programme on chronic disease management. *Australian Occupational Therapy Journal*, 60(1), 30–38. https://doi.org/10.1111/1440-1630.12008

Wolf, T. J., Baum, C. M., Lee, D., & Hammel, J. (2016). The development of the Improving Participation after Stroke Self-Management Program (IPASS): An exploratory randomized clinical study. *Topics in Stroke Rehabilitation*, 23(4), 284–292. https://doi.org/10.1080/10749357.2016.1155278

13

Occupational Therapy–Led, Educational–Behavioral Program Improves Long-Term Behavioral, Physical, and Functional Outcomes for Adults with Rheumatoid Arthritis

KRISTINE CARANDANG

[This program] highlights the importance of using educational-behavioural approaches and increasing teaching time in order to motivate, teach skills effectively and help people "change the habits and routines of a lifetime."

> HAMMOND, A., & FREEMAN, K. (2004). The long-term outcomes from a
> randomized controlled trial of an educational–behavioural joint protection
> programme for people with rheumatoid arthritis. *Clinical Rehabilitation, 18*(5),
> 520–528.

Original Paper: https://journals.sagepub.com/doi/10.1191/0269215504cr766oa

Research Question: Is an educational–behavioral joint protection program effective for those with early rheumatoid arthritis over a 4-year period?

Funding: The Arthritis Research Campaign, presently called Versus Arthritis

Year Study Began: 1995

Year Study Published: 2004

Study Location: United Kingdom

Who Was Studied: Adults who 1) were 18–65 years old; 2) had been diagnosed with rheumatoid arthritis within 5 years (groups' disease duration averaged 21 and 17.5 months); 3) experienced pain, inflammation, and functional problems in the hand and/or wrist joints; and 4) participated in the original study (Hammond & Freeman, 2001).

Who Was Excluded: Adults who had medical conditions other than rheumatoid arthritis that could affect hand function.

How Many Patients: 127

Study Overview: Study participants completed questionnaires 4 years after they were randomized into a standard education program or an educational–behavioral joint protection program (Figure 13.1).

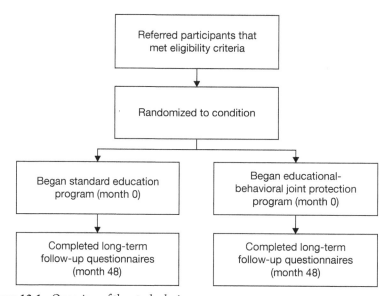

Figure 13.1. Overview of the study design.

Study Intervention: Both programs consisted of four 2-hour group sessions including patients and partners.

The educational–behavioral joint protection program was informed by the health belief model, theories of social learning, motor learning, and self-efficacy-enhancing strategies. Led by a rheumatology occupational therapist, participants practiced joint protection strategies through repetition and mental rehearsal, problem-solved potential challenges, and set goals using a provided workbook (more details in Hammond et al., 1999).

The standard education program was delivered by various rheumatology professionals who discussed and/or demonstrated topics such as medications, nutrition, exercise, and symptom management. The program included a joint protection component (approximately 2.5 hours over two sessions). Standardized for this trial, this program mimicked typical practice in the United Kingdom.

Follow-Up: 4 years (48 months)

Endpoints:

Primary outcomes:

- Hand pain experienced during moderate activity (100-mm Visual Analogue Scale)
- Use of joint protection strategies (Joint Protection Behavior Assessment [JPBA])

Secondary outcomes:

- Disease activity (symptoms, patient global rating)
- Functional assessment of activities of daily living (ADLs) and limbs (Arthritis Impact Measurement Scales 2)
- Hand grip strength
- Presence of joint deformities

RESULTS

- At 4 years post-intervention, participants in the educational–behavioral joint protection program continued to show higher use of joint protection techniques on a performance-based measure (JPBA) compared to participants in the standard education program (Table 13.1).
- For secondary measures, after 4 years, participants in the educational–behavioral joint protection program had significantly less duration (minutes) of early morning stiffness.

- After 4 years, participants in the educational–behavioral joint protection program had fewer joint deformities as evidenced by lower incidence of hand/wrist radial deviation ($p = 0.05$), wrist anterior subluxation ($p = 0.03$), and 2–5 metacarpophalangeal ulnar deviation ($p = 0.02$).
- While both groups' functional ability on ADLs worsened over time, participants in the educational–behavioral joint protection program worsened significantly less so than participants in the standard education group.
- Contrary to the 1-year post-intervention time point (Hammond & Freeman, 2001), there were no longer significant between-group differences in hand pain, overall pain, grip strength, patient-reported global disease status, or number of visits to the doctor's office after 4 years.

Table 13.1. COMPARING BASELINE AND FOLLOW-UP SCORES BETWEEN PROGRAMS (SIGNIFICANT CONSTRUCTS ONLY)

	Standard Education Program ($n = 62$)		Educational–Behavioral Joint Protection Program ($n = 65$)		p
	0 months	48 months	0 months	48 months	
Adherence to joint protection (%)	12.5 (5.0–22.5)	13.2 (6.1–25.5)	15.0 (5.0–25.0)	23.5 (12.4–44.0)	0.001
Early morning stiffness (duration in minutes)	60 (13.75–120)	60 (20.25–105)	45 (11.25–82.5)	25 (2.13–60)	0.001
Functional assessment of ADL (0 [good health status]–10 [poor health status])	1.25 (0–3.59)	1.87 (0.31–4.37)	0.8 (0–2.81)	1.25 (0–3.12)	0.04

Criticisms and Limitations:

- More data are needed to understand the effect of each intervention on pharmacological drug use.
- Alternative methods are required to measure detailed radiographic joint changes.

Other Relevant Studies and Information:

- The educational–behavioral joint protection program tested in this study was later expanded into the Lifestyle Management for Arthritis Programme (LMAP), which included other areas of self-management (e.g., pain, mood, exercise). Compared to participants in a standard education program, LMAP participants showed statistically significant improvements in pain and self-efficacy at 12-month follow-up (Hammond et al., 2008).
- Healthcare providers should consider patients' disease duration and stages of change when referring to an educational–behavioral program (Hammond & Klompenhouwer, 2005). Adults referred to a cognitive-behavioral education program within 1 month of rheumatoid arthritis diagnosis had no significant differences in physical or psychological outcomes compared to a standard education program (Freeman et al., 2002). Patients who are still managing the physical and emotional toll inherent to the early diagnosis stage may not be able to implement the lifestyle changes suggested in these programs.

Summary and Implications: At 4 years post-intervention, participants diagnosed with rheumatoid arthritis in the previous 5 years who were enrolled in an educational–behavioral joint protection program continued to use joint protection strategies and experienced long-term benefits such as less early morning stiffness, fewer deformities, and less decline in ADL functioning compared to participants in a standard education program. This study demonstrates that interventions incorporating strategies in line with behavioral, learning, and self-management theories are more effective than standard education programs delivered via mainly lecture/demonstration.

CLINICAL CASE: CONSIDERING CLIENT CONTEXT IN CHRONIC DISEASE MANAGEMENT EDUCATION

Case History

Marina (she/her), a 34-year-old Latina woman, presents to outpatient occupational therapy for hand and wrist pain related to taking care of her newborn child and with newly diagnosed rheumatoid arthritis discovered during her medical workup. She has limited understanding of her diagnosis and has questions about its long-term effects. In addition, while she has some help from her extended family, she is overwhelmed with how her functional limitations are affecting her caregiving responsibilities for her newborn and her elderly parents at home. She states, "I push through my pain but still, every step takes a lot longer than it used to. I never have time to rest." She asks how she can learn about ways to optimally function with her disease.

Suggested Answer

When considering referral to an educational–behavioral joint protection program, occupational therapists must exercise clinical reasoning by considering the client's disease duration, availability to participate in the entire program, and willingness to change health behaviors. Because the client is newly diagnosed, she is likely still learning basic information about the disease and its treatment and in initial phases of accepting its potential impact on her life. In addition, the client has concerns about her immediate responsibilities and is unlikely to be able to fully engage in the activities and practice/homework assignments involved with such a program. Therefore, it is inappropriate for an occupational therapist to refer her to this joint protection program at this time. Instead, the therapist may provide her with didactic information, collaborate to develop strategies that will help her accomplish her day-to-day tasks, and provide counseling, outside referrals, or community resources to help with her disease coping process. The therapist may also inform her of the availability of the joint protection program to revisit at a later time.

References

Freeman, K., Hammond, A. & Lincoln, N. B. (2002). Use of cognitive-behavioural arthritis education programmes in newly diagnosed rheumatoid arthritis. *Clinical Rehabilitation, 16*, 828–836.

Hammond, A., Bryan, J., & Hardy, A. (2008). Effects of a modular behavioural arthritis education programme: A pragmatic parallel-group randomized controlled trial. *Rheumatology, 47*(11), 1712–1718. https://doi.org/10.1093/rheumatology/ken380

Hammond, A., & Freeman, K. (2001). One-year outcomes of a randomized controlled trial of an educational-behavioural joint protection programme for people with rheumatoid arthritis. *Rheumatology* (Oxford, England), *40*(9), 1044–1051. https://doi.org/10.1093/rheumatology/40.9.1044

Hammond, A., & Klompenhouwer, P. (2005). Getting evidence into practice: Implementing a behavioural joint protection education programme for people with rheumatoid arthritis. *British Journal of Occupational Therapy, 68*(1), 25–33.

Hammond, A., Lincoln, N., & Sutcliffe, L. (1999). A crossover trial evaluating an educational–behavioural joint protection programme for people with rheumatoid arthritis. *Patient Education and Counseling, 37*(1), 19–32. https://doi.org/10.1016/s0738-3991(98)00093-7

14

Occupational Therapy to Improve Clinical, Behavioral, and Psychosocial Outcomes among Young Adults with Diabetes

HEATHER FRITZ

REAL Diabetes

This study provides additional evidence of the potential for OT to improve clinical and psychosocial outcomes among individuals with diabetes.

PYATAK, E. A., CARANDANG, K., VIGEN, C. L., BLANCHARD, J., DIAZ, J., CONCHA-CHAVEZ, A., SEQUEIRA, P. A., WOOD, J. R., WHITTEMORE, R., SPRUIJT-METZ, D., & PETERS, A. L. (2018). Occupational therapy intervention improves glycemic control and quality of life among young adults with diabetes: The Resilient, Empowered, Active Living with Diabetes (REAL Diabetes) randomized controlled trial. *Diabetes Care, 41*(4), 696–704.

Original Paper: https://doi.org/10.2337/dc17-1634

Research Question: Is an occupational therapy intervention to improve glycemic control and psychosocial well-being among low-income young adults with type 1 or type 2 diabetes effective?

Funding: The National Institute of Diabetes and Digestive and Kidney Diseases at the National Institutes of Health

Year Study Began: 2014

Year Study Published: 2018

Study Location: Los Angeles County, CA

Who Was Studied: Young adults ages 18-30 of low socioeconomic status who had either type 1 or type 2 diabetes for ≥ one year and who had an HbA1c of ≥ 8%.

Who Was Excluded: Pregnant individuals or those planning to become pregnant were excluded as well as individuals reporting disability limiting life expectancy, a disability that limited participation in major life activities, and previous participation in self-management interventions beyond usual care within the previous year.

How Many Patients: 81

Study Overview: Study participants were randomized to one of two groups: REAL Diabetes program or an attention-control group (Figure 14.1).

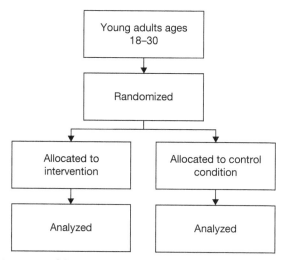

Figure 14.1. Overview of the REAL Diabetes study design.

Study Intervention: The intervention was based on the Lifestyle Redesign intervention framework and delivered by occupational therapists trained in motivational interviewing and diabetes self-management. Interventionists delivered ≥ 10 and ≤ 16 hours of treatment to participants, in their homes or community settings, over a 6-month period. The treatment consisted of seven content modules that were flexibly administered in line with participants' challenges and goals and included 1) assessment and goal-setting, 2) basic self-management knowledge and skills, 3) healthcare access and self-advocacy training, 4) establishing and maintaining health-promoting habits and routines, 5) managing social support, 6) emotional well-being, and 7) planning for long-term health.

The attention-control group received one home visit and educational materials available through the National Diabetes Education Program and MyPlate.gov. The home visit was followed by 11 biweekly phone calls during which staff asked participants if they had any questions about the materials.

Follow-Up: 6 months

Endpoints: The primary outcome was hemoglobin A1c (HbA1c). Secondary outcomes included diabetes self-care, diabetes-related quality of life (QoL), diabetes distress, depressive symptoms, medication adherence, and life satisfaction. Additional process variables included diabetes self-efficacy, diabetes knowledge, diabetes-related problem-solving, habit strength for taking medications and self-monitoring of blood glucose, and activity participation.

RESULTS

- Of the 81 participants randomized, 71 completed follow-up data collection.
- Participants were on average 22.6 ± 3.5 years old, 63% female, and 78% Hispanic and had an average HbA1c of 10.8 ± 1.9%. In total, 75% of participants had type 1 diabetes.
- Results demonstrated a significant improvement in HbA1c among intervention group (IG) participants compared with control group (CG) participants.
- IG participants had greater improvements in diabetes-related QoL compared to CG participants.
- IG participants had greater improvement in habit strength for self-monitoring of blood glucose than CG participants.
- IG participants demonstrated greater, though non-significant, improvements in all secondary outcomes with the exception of diabetes-related problem-solving compared to CG participants.

- Diabetes type, sex, ethnicity, or recruitment site did not appear to moderate treatment effects.
- Differential patterns in HbA1c trajectories showed that participants with type 1 diabetes experienced reductions in HbA1c relative to controls. Participants with type 2 diabetes experienced no significant change in HbA1c compared to controls, who exhibited large increases in HbA1c (Table 14.1).

Table 14.1. BETWEEN-GROUP DIFFERENCES IN PRIMARY AND SECONDARY STUDY OUTCOMES

Measure	Between-Group Difference in Mean Change Scores[a]	Effect Size (Cohen's d) (95% CI)	p (Two-Tailed)[b]
HbA1c	0.9	−0.5 (−0.9 to −0.1)	0.01
Diabetes-related QoL: Audit of diabetes-dependent QoL	0.5 (range: −9 to +1)	0.3 (−0.1 to 0.7)	0.04
Glucose monitoring days/week: Summary of diabetes self-care activities	0.7 (range: 0–7)	0.3 (−0.2 to 0.8)	0.37
Medication adherence days/week: Summary of diabetes self-care activities	0.2 (range: 0–7)	0.1 (−0.3 to 0.5)	0.93
Habit strength for glucose monitoring: Self-Report Behavioral Automaticity Index	2.3	0.3 (−0.2 to −0.7)	0.05
Diabetes distress: Problem Areas in Diabetes-Short Form	0.8 (range: 0–20)	−0.1 (−0.5 to 0.2)	0.26
Life satisfaction: Satisfaction with Life Scale	1.2 (range: 5–35)	0.2 (−0.2 to 0.5)	0.21
Depressive symptoms: Patient Health Questionnaire-8	0.9 (range: 0–27)	−0.2 (−0.6 to 0.2)	0.42

[a]All between-group differences favored the IG over the CG.
[b]Adjusted for baseline scores, sex, ethnicity, recruitment site, diabetes type, and socioeconomic status. All p values are two-sided.

Criticisms and Limitations: The study was limited by the small, non-representative (e.g., predominantly Hispanic) sample and insufficient statistical power to examine mediation or moderation or definitively analyze secondary outcomes. Due to the lack of long-term follow-up, it is unclear whether treatment effects were maintained after cessation of the intervention.

Other Relevant Studies and Information:

- A hybrid effectiveness-implementation study examining the feasibility of implementing REAL Diabetes into a primary care setting indicated improvements in HbA1c, blood pressure, health behaviors, and overall health status for those receiving the occupational therapy treatment (Pyatak et al., 2019).
- A culturally tailored occupational therapy group intervention for Mexican Americans that addressed participants' diabetes acceptance and healthcare beliefs as well as the need to change habits, develop goals, and advocate for one's needs led to improved empowerment, self-efficacy, and lowered HbA1c levels (Haltiwanger, 2012).
- A scoping review of interventions designed to help individuals develop new habits or weaken existing habits provided evidence that habit formation treatments can result in habit formation and change. Few studies, however, have shown how changes in habit lead to changes in clinical outcomes (Fritz et al., 2020).

Summary and Implications: An occupational therapy program for young adults with diabetes had favorable effects on blood glucose control and diabetes-related QoL. The study results support the benefit of occupational therapy as part of an interdisciplinary care team to improve diabetes-related health and well-being.

CLINICAL CASE: DIABETES MANAGEMENT IN A PRIMARY CARE CLINIC

Case History

An occupational therapist (OT) working at a primary care clinic has been asked to provide an evidence-based intervention for individuals with diabetes. The clinic has an increased number of young adult clients with diabetes who continue to struggle with diabetes self-management (DSM), despite receiving basic diabetes education and a consultation with a nutritionist. The clinic is hoping to develop a program that will help clients develop healthy habits and routines, better navigate healthcare access, advocate for their needs, and maintain their emotional well-being and QoL.

Based on the REAL Diabetes study, what should the OT do to address this need?

Suggested Answer

Evidence would support the OT creating a program based on the REAL Diabetes study to help clients develop healthy habits and maintain overall health and QoL. The OT knows that didactic education alone is insufficient to support the complexities of DSM. The OT should begin by assessing the clients DSM goals and delivering DSM knowledge and skills relevant to the client's unique needs. The OT should also include education and training in how to access and navigate healthcare to meet short- and long-term care needs, strategies to develop healthy habits and maintain emotional well-being, and training in self-advocacy. A program such as this would improve DSM and promote health and QoL.

References

Fritz, H., Hu, Y. L., Gahman, K., Almacen, C., & Ottolini, J. (2020). Intervention to modify habits: A scoping review. *OTJR: Occupation, Participation and Health, 40*(2), 99–112. https://doi.org/10.1177/1539449219876877

Haltiwanger, E. P. (2012). Effect of a group adherence intervention for Mexican-American older adults with type 2 diabetes. *American Journal of Occupational Therapy, 66*(4), 447–454. https://doi.org/10.5014/ajot.2012.004457

Pyatak, E., King, M., Vigen, C. L., Salazar, E., Diaz, J., Schepens Niemiec, S. L., Blanchard, J., Jordan, M. K., Banerjee, J., & & Shukla, J. (2019). Addressing diabetes in primary care: Hybrid effectiveness–implementation study of Lifestyle Redesign® occupational therapy. *American Journal of Occupational Therapy, 73*(5), 7305185020p1–7305185020p12.

SECTION 3

Work and Industry

The term "occupation" is most associated with one's job or employment, leading to a question that is often asked of occupational therapy (OT) practitioners: "Do you help people find jobs?" While it may be easy to immediately dismiss this as an inaccurate description of the profession, some OT practitioners do assist in identifying and selecting employment opportunities for individuals with varied physical, psychological, and social functional capacities. In fact, work and employment was a key construct upon which the profession was founded as early occupational therapists supported soldiers to re-engage in their jobs after injury. "Work" is considered one of the core areas of occupation within the profession that incorporates employment interests and pursuits, employment seeking and acquisition, job performance and maintenance, retirement preparation and adjustment, and volunteer exploration and participation (American Occupational Therapy Association, 2020).

OT practitioners are unique from other professionals who engage within the area of work and industry as they use a holistic lens and consider the numerous transactions among the complex systems that make up the worker, the work, and the work environment. Traditional engagement within this area of practice involves the prevention of musculoskeletal disorders through occupational analyses and ergonomic interventions, rehabilitation for work-related injuries through clinic-based interventions, and support for general physical health and mental well-being through services at the work site (e.g., interpersonal skills training, time management). Beyond these work-centric services, OT practitioners are key members of the healthcare team who have the training and skills to support return to work following a major medical event, such as a stroke, traumatic brain injury, or spinal cord injury, and can provide vocational services to promote gainful employment for individuals with chronic or stigmatized conditions that may impact functional or social engagement in the workplace, such as diabetes, fibromyalgia, and mental health conditions.

OT practitioners play a vital role in supporting employment and well-being for an increasingly diverse workforce. For example, neuro-diverse individuals are a key demographic of workers that OT practitioners are well suited to support through the application of a person–occupation–environment perspective as a means for ensuring successful gainful employment. Existing published evidence is primarily limited to ways in which the profession supports individuals with varied functional abilities. There is a need for more research and practice-based evidence that describes the role of OT practitioners in supporting equity, inclusion, access, and positive workplace climates and cultures for other populations historically marginalized due to their race, ethnicity, gender, age, sexual orientation, mental health status, neurodiversity, etc. Given the use of a holistic lens, OT practitioners are well positioned to be leaders as workplace health and worker well-being paradigms shift to account for the lived experiences of workers both within and outside the workplace (Chari et al., 2018).

The studies in this section have been selected to highlight the broad scope of OT in the work and industry area of practice. The first two studies focus on the traditional core practice areas of ergonomics (Feingold & Jacobs) and rehabilitation of work-related musculoskeletal disorders (Hardison & Roll). The third study (Holmlund et al.) describes the importance of considering return-to-work during the acute and post-acute rehabilitation process as well as after discharge from traditional clinical rehabilitation for individuals with life-altering medical conditions, such as spinal cord injury. In addition to those with physical disabilities, the Kielhofner et al. study demonstrates how a human occupation perspective can be deployed relative to vocational rehabilitation for individuals with other chronic conditions. This section concludes with an example of the emerging role for occupational therapists in supporting inclusion and access by highlighting a study that considers how workplace environments can be maximized to ensure success of individuals with autism in the workforce (Pfeiffer et al.). Taken together, these studies represent current perspectives and future opportunities for OT practice within work and industry.

Who Was Studied: Seventh-grade students who wear backpacks defined as a bag carried on the back with two shoulder straps. The sample included nine female and eight male children aged 12 and 13 years (average 12.7 years); 83.4% were Caucasian, and 16.6% were Asian.

Who Was Excluded: Children who did not own or use a backpack, and those children unable to attend all three research sessions.

How Many Participants: 17

Study Overview: See Figure 15.1.

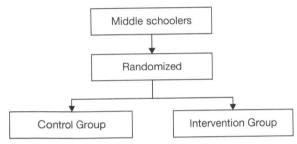

Figure 15.1. Overview of the study design.

Study Intervention: The study intervention consisted of a 30-minute educational video on proper backpack wearing and posture. The video contains four rules of backpack wearing: "Choose right, pack right, lift right, wear right." Study personnel provided demonstrations and hands-on application of the educational material. Participants were also asked to list the content of their backpacks and questioned why they were not using the waist-belt of their backpacks. Participants were asked to implement proper backpack wearing for the next week. Participants in the control group did not receive any study-related intervention but were able to watch a recording of the intervention session at the conclusion of the study.

Follow-Up: Initial follow-up measures were conducted 1 week after the intervention. There was no long-term follow-up.

Endpoints:

Primary outcomes:

- Postures while carrying a backpack were measured using anatomical markers in four conditions: without a bag, with a bag using one

---

References

American Occupational Therapy Association. (2020). Occupational therapy practice framework: Domain and process—fourth edition. *American Journal of Occupational Therapy*, 74(Supplement 2), Article 7412410010. https://doi.org/10.5014/ajot.2020.74S2001

Chari, R., Chang, C. C., Sauter, S. L., Sayers, E. L. P., Cerully, J. L., Schulte, P., Schill, A. L., & Uscher-Pines, L. (2018). Expanding the paradigm of occupational safety and health a new framework for worker well-being. *Journal of Occupational and Environmental Medicine*, 60(7), 589.

15

Injury Prevention through Ergonomic Assessment, Education, and Intervention

Healthy Backpack Wearing in School-Aged Children

YOKO E. FUKUMURA AND SHAWN C. ROLL

> 87.5% of the intervention group members proceeded to continue wearing the backpack properly . . . since the intervention, two participants reported that wearing the backpack properly resulted in less pain in their back, four participants reported that they experienced less pressure and pain on their shoulders, and one participant reported that she experienced less strain in her neck.
>
> FEINGOLD, A. J., & JACOBS, K. (2002). The effect of
> education on backpack wearing and posture in
> a middle school population. *Work, 18*(3), 287–294.

Original Paper: https://content.iospress.com/articles/work/wor00240

Research Question: What effect does ergonomics education on proper ba
pack wearing have on posture and appropriate backpack-wearing techniqu
middle school children?

Funding: Not available

Year Study Began: Not available

Year Study Published: 2002

Study Location: Andover, MA (Andover West Middle School)

strap, with a bag using two straps, and with a bag in the participant's preferred method. Change in posture was defined as lateral or forward flexion in individual joints and was calculated using AngleCalc, a computer program written by the Boston University computer science department.
- Backpack weight was obtained by weighing students with and without backpacks. The two measurements were used to calculate the percentage of body weight being carried in the backpack.

Secondary outcomes:

- Use of backpack waist-belt.
- Participant self-report on impact of education on musculoskeletal discomfort.

RESULTS

- Of the 17 participants, 13 completed all sessions of the study, with primary dropout occurring in the control group.
- The intervention group had a smaller average degree of absolute change in lateral joint angles from no backpack to wearing a backpack with two straps and with the participant's preferred way. However, no statistically significant difference was found in backpack-wearing posture after education.
- There was a slight decrease in backpack weight from the first to the last session from 15.2% of body weight to 14.4%, after backpack weights were normalized.
- Participants in the intervention group self-reported a decrease in pain and pressure after education.
- At the beginning of the study, none of the participants wore the waist-belt of their backpacks. In the intervention group, six out of the seven who had backpacks with waist-belts started wearing them. In the control group, none of the participants used the waist-belts.

Criticisms and Limitations: This study was an experimental pilot trial that included a small convenience sample. This sampling coupled with differential attrition confounded interpretation of inconclusive results due to limited statistical power and reduced generalizability of the findings. The study did not have long-term follow-up to understand the sustained impact of education on middle school children's backpack-wearing posture and musculoskeletal comfort.

Other Relevant Studies and Information:

- Ergonomic education and on-site intervention provided by occupational therapists have been shown to be effective in various populations, such as to improve posture and workstation design in microscope workers (Darragh et al., 2008) and to increase awareness of posture and work practices in radiologic professionals (Fisher, 2015).
- Occupational therapists can apply their holistic approach to enhance ergonomic features and support healthy human engagement as part of product design, such as wheelchair cushions for postural support (Timm & Samuelsson, 2016), computer setup and equipment for individuals with various medical conditions (Baker et al., 2012; Liu et al., 2019), and development of artificial intelligence within the built environment to promote productivity, health, and well-being in office workplaces (Aryal et al., 2019).
- Occupational therapists themselves are at risk for developing work-related musculoskeletal injury (Dyrkacz et al., 2012), with a study showing an annual rate of 16.5 injuries per 100 full-time occupational therapists (Darragh et al., 2009). There is a need to address injury prevention by foregrounding ergonomics in occupational therapy education (Strong et al., 2003) and as part of training in safe patient handling in order to prevent workplace injury in occupational therapists (Darragh et al., 2009).

Summary and Implications: This study demonstrated how education on proper backpack wearing and posture can impact health behavior in middle school children. Implementing effective ergonomic education is essential to preventing musculoskeletal discomfort and injury, an important concept that can be applied across the life span beginning with reduction of poor habits and maladaptive physical postures in growing children. This work led to the founding of the American Occupational Therapy Association's annual National School Backpack Awareness Day and the development of numerous resources for therapists, parents, teachers, and children to support positive musculoskeletal health.

CLINICAL CASE: TREATING A MIDDLE SCHOOL VIOLIST'S UPPER BODY PAIN

Case History

Eloise (she/her), a 12-year-old girl, is referred to occupational therapy due to neck and back pain. She plays viola in the school orchestra. She lives close to school and walks for 15 minutes each way while carrying a backpack and her viola. Due to her pain, she is upset and embarrassed about not being able to play viola for the entirety of the 1-hour-long orchestra rehearsals in school. She has also been unable to participate in some activities during her physical education class in school. What should the occupational therapist focus on?

Suggested Answer

This study highlights the impact of education on proper backpack wearing and posture on musculoskeletal comfort. Education on the four rules of backpack wearing and hands-on practice may help to decrease Eloise's spinal load during the daily commute. The occupational therapist may also discuss the contents of the backpack to decrease the amount carried every day. Additionally, posture during other activities such as attending class and playing viola are important to consider so that she can continue to engage in her meaningful occupations. Using resources from the American Occupational Therapy Association's National School Backpack Awareness Day, the therapist may also contact the school with an offer to set up an annual program for all students in conjunction with other national events each fall (American Occupational Therapy Association, n.d.).

References

American Occupational Therapy Association. (n.d.). *Backpack day handouts, artwork, and video*. Retrieved June 21, 2022, from https://www.aota.org/~/media/Corporate/Files/Backpack/Backpack-Awareness-Day-Media-Advisory.docx

Aryal, A., Becerik-Gerber, B., Anselmo, F., Roll, S. C., & Lucas, G. M. (2019). Smart desks to promote comfort, health, and productivity in offices: A vision for future workplaces. Frontiers in Built Environment, 5, Article 76. https://doi.org/10.3389/fbuil.2019.00076

Baker, N. A., Aufman, E. L., & Poole, J. L. (2012). Computer use problems and accommodation strategies at work and home for people with systemic sclerosis: A needs assessment. *American Journal of Occupational Therapy, 66*(3), 368–375. https://doi.org/10.5014/ajot.2012.003467

Darragh, A. R., Harrison, H., & Kenny, S. (2008). Effect of an ergonomics intervention on workstations of microscope workers. *American Journal of Occupational Therapy*, 62(1), 61–69. https://doi.org/10.5014/ajot.62.1.61

Darragh, A. R., Huddleston, W., & King, P. (2009). Work-related musculoskeletal injuries and disorders among occupational and physical therapists. *American Journal of Occupational Therapy*, 63(3), 351–362. https://doi.org/10.5014/ajot.63.3.351

Dyrkacz, A. P., Mak, L. Y. M., & Heck, C. S. (2012). Work-related injuries in Canadian occupational therapy practice. *Canadian Journal of Occupational Therapy*, 79(4), 237–247. https://doi.org/10.2182/cjot.2012.79.4.5

Fisher, T. F. (2015). Radiologic and sonography professionals' ergonomics: An occupational therapy intervention for preventing work injuries. *Journal of Diagnostic Medical Sonography*, 31(3), 137–147. https://doi.org/10.1177/8756479315580020

Liu, S. Q., Zhang, J. C., & Zhu, R. (2019). A wearable human motion tracking device using micro flow sensor incorporating with micro accelerometer. *IEEE Transactions on Biomedical Engineering*, 67(4), 940–948. https://doi.org/10.1109/tbme.2019.2924689

Strong, S., Baptiste, S., & Salvatori, P. (2003). Learning from today's clinicians in vocational practice to educate tomorrow's therapists. *Canadian Journal of Occupational Therapy*, 70(1), 11–20. https://doi.org/10.1177/000841740307000103

Timm, M., & Samuelsson, K. (2016). Wheelchair seating: A study on the healthy elderly. *Scandinavian Journal of Occupational Therapy*, 23(6), 458–466. https://doi.org/10.3109/11038128.2016.1152297

16

Occupational Rehabilitation for Work-Related Musculoskeletal Disorders

JEFF SNODGRASS

Clients who received work simulation as a part of rehabilitation were 6.4 times as likely to succeed than those who did not receive work simulation ... findings highlight the importance of maximizing therapeutic intensity in the treatment of [work-related musculoskeletal disorders] within occupational rehabilitation programs.

HARDISON, M. E., & ROLL, S. C. (2017). Factors associated with success in an occupational rehabilitation program for work-related musculoskeletal disorders. *American Journal of Occupational Therapy, 71*(1), 7101190040p1–7101190040p8.

Original Paper: https://doi.org/10.5014/ajot.2016.023200

Research Questions: What are the client and program factors that predict success for clients in a general occupational rehabilitation program (i.e., work conditioning) and in a comprehensive occupational rehabilitation program (i.e., work hardening)? Is the presence of interventions in the area of occupations and activities via simulated work tasks associated with successful outcomes?

Funding: The National Institutes of Health Rehabilitation Research Career Development Program.

Year Study Began: 2003

Year Study Published: 2017

Study Location: Los Angeles, CA

Who Was Studied: Clients who had received either general or comprehensive occupational rehabilitation at a Commission on Accreditation of Rehabilitation Facilities–accredited outpatient facility in the Midwestern United States between 2003 and 2011. The clients included as part of both programs were predominantly male, unskilled laborers with an average age of 42.6 years.

Who Was Excluded: Clients who had previously participated in an occupational rehabilitation program.

How Many Patients: 166

Study Overview: See Figure 16.1.

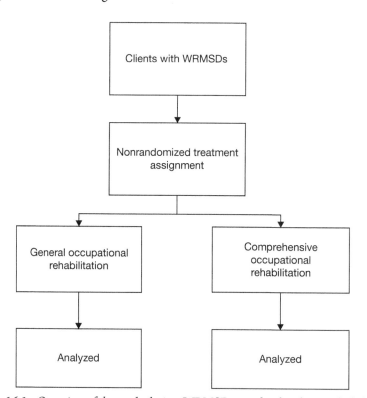

Figure 16.1. Overview of the study design. WRMSD = work-related musculoskeletal disorder.

Study Intervention: The clinic provided both general and comprehensive occupational rehabilitation programs (i.e., work conditioning and work hardening, respectively). The general occupational rehabilitation program was provided by occupational therapy with a goal of improving general physical tolerance and endurance necessary for a client to be successful in returning to part-time work (up to 20 hours/week). In contrast, the comprehensive occupational rehabilitation program was an individually tailored program provided to clients with complex cases who required interdisciplinary care (e.g., occupational therapy, physical therapy, psychology, dietetics, nursing) and individualized, intensive rehabilitation to improve tolerance for returning to full-time work at 40 hours/week.

Follow-Up: Not available

Endpoints: Primary Outcome: Successful return to work as defined by one of the following at the time of discharge:
- returned to work at any job
- cleared by a physician to return to work and initiated a job search process
- progressed to additional services within a vocational rehabilitation plan meant to support obtaining employment (e.g., vocational counseling, specialized technical training)

RESULTS

Of the clients in the general occupational rehabilitation program, 81% (77 of 95) achieved a successful return to work outcome. Successful discharge status was noted for 68% (48 of 71) of clients who received the comprehensive occupational rehabilitation program, a significantly lower success rate than the general program ($p = 0.047$). Key findings include:
- No difference was found in gender, labor type, marital status, injury type, age, number of diagnoses, lost time from work, or pain between clients with different program success outcomes.
- The frequency of successful return to work outcome was higher for clients who received work simulation versus those who received rehabilitation without work simulation and attended more, and longer, sessions ($p < 0.001$).
- Session length was highly correlated with work simulation ($r = 0.690$, $p < 0.001$), moderately correlated with number of sessions ($r = 0.394$, $p < 0.001$), and highly skewed toward 4 hours.

- Female clients were less likely to succeed in work conditioning than male clients (odds ratio = 0.186, p = 0.033), and each additional session attended increased a client's chance of success by 29% (p = 0.001).
- Clients who received work simulation as a part of their work conditioning rehabilitation were 6.4 times as likely to succeed than those who did not receive work simulation (p = 0.014).
- Every additional hour per session spent in work hardening increased the likelihood of a successful discharge status by nearly 3.5 times (p < 0.001) (Table 16.1).

TABLE 16.1. FINAL ODDS RATIOS FOR VARIABLES PREDICTING POSITIVE OUTCOMES OF GENERAL AND COMPREHENSIVE OCCUPATIONAL REHABILITATION

Variable	Odds Ratio	p
General occupational rehabilitation (n = 95)		
Gender: female	0.186	0.033
Number of sessions	1.292	0.001
Work simulation: yes	6.369	0.014
Comprehensive occupational rehabilitation (n = 71)		
Session length: hours	3.491	<0.001

Criticisms and Limitations: The study's primary limitations are due to the retrospective design, limiting the ability to make causal inferences, and sample size, limiting statistical power. Additionally, the design of the study and limited access to additional key variables including actual return to work status limit the analysis to an exploratory model to identify potential predictors of successful return to work.

Other Relevant Studies and Information:

- This study demonstrates the importance of occupation and activity interventions, in this case simulated work activities, as a component of the rehabilitation process, which has been noted as an important need within other systematic reviews of occupational therapy interventions for individuals with musculoskeletal conditions (Roll & Hardison, 2017).
- Findings from a systematic review of the literature related to effective occupational therapy interventions in rehabilitation of individuals with work-related low back injuries strongly suggest that, for interventions to be effective, occupational therapy practitioners should use a holistic,

client-centered approach. The research supports the importance for occupational therapy practitioners to consider multiple strategies for addressing clients' needs. Specifically, interventions for individuals with low back injuries and illnesses should incorporate a biopsychosocial, client-centered approach (Snodgrass, 2011)

- A randomized controlled trial examined the effects of an inpatient multicomponent occupational rehabilitation program compared to less comprehensive outpatient rehabilitation. This study provided no support that the more comprehensive inpatient multicomponent occupational rehabilitation program reduced sickness absence compared to the outpatient rehabilitation program (Aasdahl et al., 2018).

Summary and Implications: The findings of this study indicate new factors associated with success in occupational rehabilitation, specifically highlighting the importance of intensity of therapy (i.e., session length and number of sessions) and occupation-based activities for this population.

CLINICAL CASE: RETURNING A CLIENT TO WORK USING AN OCCUPATIONAL REHABILITATION APPROACH

Case History

Mai (she/her), a 50-year-old woman working in the shipping department of an online retailer, suffered a work-related herniated nucleus pulposus requiring surgical repair. The surgeon has referred the client postoperatively to receive inpatient rehabilitation to prepare her for a full return to work in her preinjury job as a shipping clerk. The workers' compensation case manager contacted the supervising occupational therapist at a regional inpatient rehabilitation hospital regarding whether the facility provides a focused occupational rehabilitation program. The facility has experienced a significant increase in admissions for individuals with work-related musculoskeletal disorders of the back and extremities. How should the supervising occupational therapist respond?

Suggested Answer

The evidence would suggest that intensity of an occupational rehabilitation program for individuals with work-related musculoskeletal disorders is important, and occupations and activities intervention strategies may be a strong, active component related to success in occupational rehabilitation. The supervising occupational therapist should inform the case manager that best practices suggest the importance of intensity (i.e., session length and number of sessions) of therapy. The supervising occupational therapist should also inform the case manager that the facility will emphasize an interdisciplinary approach to the client's rehabilitation (e.g., occupational therapy, physical therapy, psychology, dietetics, nursing) with a focus on work simulation and longer individual sessions.

References

Aasdahl, L., Pape, K., Vasseljen, O., Johnsen, R., Gismervik, S., Halsteinli, V., Fleten, N., Nielsen, C. V., & Fimland, M. S. (2018). Effect of inpatient multicomponent occupational rehabilitation versus less comprehensive outpatient rehabilitation on sickness absence in persons with musculoskeletal- or mental health disorders: A randomized clinical trial. *Journal of Occupational Rehabilitation, 28*(1), 170–179. https://doi.org/10.1007/s10926-017-9708-z

Roll, S. C., & Hardison, M. E. (2017). Effectiveness of occupational therapy interventions for adults with musculoskeletal conditions of the forearm, wrist, and hand: A systematic review. *American Journal of Occupational Therapy, 71,* 7101180010p1–7101180010p12. https://doi.org/10.5014/ajot.2017.023234

Snodgrass, J. (2011). Effective occupational therapy interventions in the rehabilitation of individuals with work-related low back injuries and illnesses: A systematic review. *American Journal of Occupational Therapy, 65,* 37–43. https://doi.org/10.5014/ajot.2011.09187

17

Return to Work after Spinal Cord Injury

A Need for Early, Individually Tailored Rehabilitation Care

ALIX G. SLEIGHT

Persons who have no higher education or lack viable employment to return to after spinal cord injury (SCI) seem to be vulnerable in return to work. Early and timely interventions tailored to the person's interests and competencies, in which the rehabilitation team has a distinct coordinating role, are thus critical in return to work.

> HOLMLUND, L., GUIDETTI, S., ERIKSSON, G., & ASABA, E. (2017). Return to work in the context of everyday life 7–11 years after spinal cord injury—A follow-up study. *Disability and Rehabilitation, 40*(24), 2875–2883.

Original Paper: https://www.tandfonline.com/doi/abs/10.1080/09638288.2017.1362597

Research Question: How do young adults experience return to work in the context of everyday life after spinal cord injury (SCI)?

Funding: The Doctoral School in Health Care Sciences at Karolinska Institutet, Norrbacka-Eugenia Foundation, Neuro Sweden, Spinalis Foundation, and the Swedish Association of Occupational Therapists

Year Study Began: 2008

Year Study Published: 2017

Study Location: Stockholm, Sweden

Who Was Studied: Individuals with traumatic SCI were included. Participants were Swedish, 20–34 years of age, 7–11 years post-injury, and had not yet returned to work. Four individuals had paraplegia, and four had tetraplegia.

Who Was Excluded: Individuals were excluded from the study if they had received occupational therapy services from the first author and/or if they had a psychiatric diagnosis as defined in the Axis I and Axis II *Diagnostic and Statistical Manual of Mental Disorders*-IV.

How Many Participants: 8

Study Overview: This qualitative study involved in-depth interviews (one to three per participant) lasting 45–120 minutes and supplementary observations (either none or one per participant). A narrative approach was used, and open-ended questions were posed to elicit storied descriptions involving work. Conceptual areas explored included patterns of everyday life, the meaning of work, experience and expectations of return to work, and support in the return to work process. Observations included situations and places where participants spent significant time during the day (e.g., home, studio, coffee shop). Data were analyzed using iterative thematic analysis of narratives.

Study Intervention: Not applicable.

Follow-Up: Not applicable.

RESULTS

Five main themes emerged from the analysis. These themes generally revolved around experiences of return to work in the context of everyday life.
- *Negotiating the possibilities of working*: Participants described trying to juggle priorities in their everyday lives (e.g., self-care, parenting roles) with the desire to return to work.
- *Hope for future work tempered with concern*: Participants felt optimistic about returning to work eventually but expressed fears about fitting in to the labor market and finding a position that suited their interests and competencies.

- *Education as a possible path to employment*: Participants described the nuances of pursuing education or additional training as an entryway to return to work. However, education was often described as a calculated economic risk.
- *Paths toward return to work in the light of unmet support*: Participants discussed reaching out for support from various stakeholders (e.g., government agencies) when looking for work. They often did not receive the support they needed, resulting in either resignation or a need to find solutions independently.
- *Unpaid occupations grounded in interest and competence*: Participants sometimes replaced traditional paid work with involvement in valued unpaid occupations (e.g., computer engineering, writing, artwork). Some anticipated that these occupations could open possibilities for future employment.

Most participants reported transitioning to a life without work, though for many there was still hope for future employment. Return to work was experienced as constantly needing to be negotiated in the context of everyday life. Participants reported many common experiences, but there were differences between those who had found work and those who had not returned to work post-injury. Rehabilitation programs have the potential to support individuals seeking to return to work after SCI by coordinating both medical and return-to-work needs during the process of rehabilitation. Close cooperation between vocational and clinical rehabilitation—with an emphasis on the individual's employment preferences—is warranted in this population.

Criticisms and Limitations: As a small, qualitative study, this work has limited generalizability. In addition, the participants were primarily male, resulting in a lack of representation of the experiences of women in returning to work after SCI.

Other Relevant Studies and Information:

- This study was used as a foundation for the development of an intervention for return to work in individuals with SCI in Sweden. The intervention, "Re-Work-SCI," develops an individualized, occupation-based plan for returning to work for participants, facilitates decision-making, and builds trust in the return-to-work process after SCI (Holmlund et al., 2020).

- This work has also been used in the development of occupational science scholarship critically evaluating the concepts of return to work and unemployment. Specifically, work by Asaba et al. (2020) investigates ways in which narrow conceptualizations of "work" can restrict the possibilities of work-related occupations.
- This work reflects a push for early, personally tailored care coordination for individuals with other chronic conditions such as cancer to facilitate successful return to work (e.g., Newman et al., 2019; Stout et al., 2019).
- Finally, this work informs scholarship about the role of occupational therapy in other chronic conditions such as stroke. These studies call for the integration of well-coordinated and optimally timed return-to-work programs into rehabilitation (e.g., Scott & Bondoc, 2018).

Summary and Implications: This qualitative study investigated how young adults experience return to work in the context of everyday life after SCI. Return to work was experienced as constantly needing to be negotiated in the context of everyday life. Participants reported many common experiences, but there were differences between those who had found work and those who had not returned to work post-injury. People without higher education and those who lack viable employment to return to after SCI were found to be more vulnerable in return to work. Importantly, early and timely rehabilitation interventions tailored to unique patient interests and competencies may be critical in successful return to work following a traumatic injury or medical condition.

CLINICAL CASE: RETURN TO WORK AFTER SCI

Case History

Jacob (he/him), a 26-year-old man with a complete lumbar SCI resulting in paraplegia, is referred to occupational therapy for return to work after his motor vehicle accident. Prior to his injury, he worked as a landscaper part time while pursuing graduate education in computer programming. His undergraduate degree is in mathematics. Jacob lives alone with his German shepherd and enjoys playing online video games with friends in his spare time. Based on the results of this qualitative study, what are the most important considerations for this patient?

Suggested Answer

Holmlund et al. found that individuals without higher education or a clear vocation to return to were particularly vulnerable to difficulties with returning to work after SCI. Therefore, two key considerations would be Jacob's level of education and vocation before the motor vehicle accident. Jacob will be unable to return to his previous work as a landscaper due to the physical demands of the job. However, he has an undergraduate degree in mathematics and had completed several credits toward a graduate degree in computer programming prior to his injury. These elements of his occupational history will bolster his chances of returning to work. The occupational therapist should work with Jacob to determine whether he wants to pursue his previous career path and, if so, support him in obtaining any necessary accommodations for the completion of his graduate degree. In addition, rehabilitation after SCI should focus on how return to work fits with the complex fabric of preexisting roles, routines, interests, and competencies. After completing Jacob's occupational profile to determine his unique everyday activities, strengths, challenges, and goals, the occupational therapist should determine how a return to a role as a graduate student would integrate with Jacob's additional roles (e.g., caregiver for his pet, online gaming enthusiast). Initiating return-to-work therapy as early as possible for Jacob would be key, and coordination with other healthcare professionals and support networks would also be instrumental in his successful return to employment.

References

Asaba, E., Aldrich, R. M., Gabrielsson, H., Ekstam, L., & Farias, L. (2020). Challenging conceptualisations of work: Revisiting contemporary experiences of return to work and unemployment. *Journal of Occupational Science, 23*, 1–4.

Holmlund, L., Guidetti, S., Hultling, C., Seiger, A., Eriksson, G., & Asaba, E. (2020). Evaluating the feasibility of ReWork-SCI: A person-centred intervention for return-to-work after spinal cord injury. *BMJ Open, 10*, Article e036000. https://doi.org/10.1136/bmjopen-2019-036000

Newman, R. M., Alfano, C. M., Radomski, M. V., Pergolotti, M., Wolf, T. J., Sleight, A. G., Bryant, A. L., Voelbel, G. T., de Moor, J. S., Nitkin, R., Daniels, E., Braveman, B., Walker, R. K., Williams, G. R., Winters-Stone, K. M., Cheville, A. L., Campbell, S. E., Lawlor, M. C., King, A. A., . . . Lyons, K. D. (2019). Catalyzing research to optimize cancer survivors' participation in work and life roles. *OTJR: Occupation, Participation and Health, 39*(4), 189–196. https://doi.org/10.1177/1539449219844749

Scott, S. L., & Bondoc, S. (2018). Return to work after stroke: A survey of occupational therapy practice patterns. *Occupational Therapy in Health Care, 32*(3), 195–215. https://doi.org/10.1080/07380577.2018.1491083

Stout, N. L., Sleight, A., Pfeiffer, D., Galantino, M. L., & deSouza, B. (2019). Promoting assessment and management of function through navigation: Opportunities to bridge oncology and rehabilitation systems of care. *Supportive Care in Cancer, 27*, 4497–4505. https://doi.org/10.1007/s00520-019-04741-0

18

Emerging Occupational Therapy Practice for Inclusive Work Transition and Vocational Programming

SELENA WASHINGTON AND LISA JAEGERS

Given the multiple impairments and social problems of this cohort of persons with AIDS, the Employment Options program appears to have achieved the rate of success as good as that reported in the literature for well-developed programs.

KIELHOFNER, G., BRAVEMAN, B., FINLAYSON, M., PAUL-WARD, A., GOLDBAUM, L., & GOLDSTEIN, K. (2004). Outcomes of a vocational program for persons with AIDS. *American Journal of Occupational Therapy, 58*(1), 64–72.

Original Paper: https://doi.org/10.5014/ajot.58.1.64

Research Questions: What was the rate of completion for an occupational therapy–based vocational training program for individuals with AIDS? What was the rate of successful return to work, school, or volunteering for clients who completed the vocational program? What initial participant characteristics were the best predictors of program completion and successful program outcomes?

Funding: The AIDS Foundation of Chicago, Rehabilitation Services Administration, US Department of Education

Year Study Began: Not available

Year Study Published: 2004

Study Location: Chicago, IL

Who Was Studied: Adult men and women with a medical diagnosis of HIV/ AIDS and an expressed desire to achieve employment.

Who Was Excluded: Participants were not accepted into the program if they did not demonstrate an interest in exploring the possibility of achieving employment, were unable to participate in a structured community-based program, or were actively abusing drugs/alcohol.

How Many Participants: 129

Study Overview: Study participants were followed at four time points to assess completion of the program and participation in work pursuits (Figure 18.1).

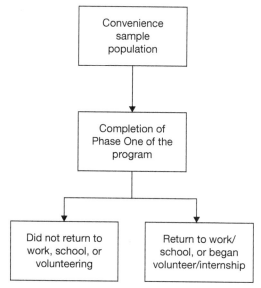

Figure 18.1. Overview of the study design.

Study Intervention: This intervention study examined the outcomes of the Employment Options Program, a four-phase service program based on the Model of Human Occupation development continuum of volition, habituation, and performance capacity (Kielhofner, 2002). The program's staff consisted of two occupational therapists responsible for the individual and group intervention throughout the program's phases and a vocational specialist who provided workplace training and services.

Participants who were enrolled in the first phase ($n = 90$) completed a comprehensive self-assessment and refinement of vocational choice and identified relevant work skills and habits to inform the return to work of the Employment Options Program. During this phase, participants attended group sessions to address the logistics of returning to work and individual sessions designed to support the development of the daily habits needed in a vocational role. Phase two provided opportunities to address and cope with the challenges associated with working, through confidence-building activities employed to assist the participants with identifying their values and strengths and to manage the routine of working. Phase three supported successful employment through participant placement in paid jobs developed by the program or by employment referrals. During this phase, interventions such as job analysis, modifications, and participant/employer coaching were provided. The fourth phase sustained participant employment through ongoing periodic workplace training and services, provided by the program staff as needed.

Follow-Up: Follow-up sessions were conducted at 6, 12, 18, and 24 months after enrollment and collection of baseline data.

Endpoints: Successful participant outcomes were defined as regularly volunteering, being in school, or achieving employment at any of the follow-up points.

Occupational Performance History Interview-II (OPHI-II) interviews were used to develop narrative slopes to visually portray how the respondent's life had unfolded (Braveman & Helfrich, 2001; Kielhofner et al., 1997). Progressive slopes indicated a clear and sustained upward turn (i.e., change for the better); stable narratives were characterized by patterns of minimal change over time. Regressive slopes indicated a downward turn (i.e., change for the worse) in life.

RESULTS

- Demographic characteristics of the 129 participants included the following: 82% male, 44% African American, 85% education of high school or greater, 13% history of incarceration, 44% history of substance misuse, 84% history of mental illness, and 26% additional physical diagnoses.

- Program completion rates: 30% left the program before finishing phase one (not completed) and 90 participants completed the program, with 67% ($n = 60$) achieving a successful outcome. Persons with regressive narratives failed to complete the first phase of the program at a rate more than twice that of persons with progressive narratives.
- Successful outcomes: achieved employment ($n = 50$), returned to school ($n = 2$), participated in a volunteer position or internship ($n = 8$).
- Characteristics associated with successful program outcomes:
  - Compared to persons with a regressive slope, persons with a progressive slope were more likely to experience a positive outcome.
  - Persons with a history of mental illness were more likely to have a successful outcome compared to those without a history.

Criticisms and Limitations: Key limitations in this study include use of a convenience sample and lack of a control group for comparing the outcomes of the study, which weakens the generalizability of findings.

Other Relevant Studies and Information:

- A collaborative job-matching process allows stakeholders to consider a multitude of inputs for determining job matches. There's an opportunity for occupational therapy practitioners to improve positive outcomes of job-matching by streamlining practices through improved consistency and defining outcomes of interest (Persch, Cleary et al., 2015).
- This study incorporates multiple measures of work and occupational participation developed by occupational therapists that may be useful in assessments for intervention planning, including the OPHI-II (Kielhofner et al., 1997), the Worker Role Interview (Velozo et al., 1998), and the Occupational Self Assessment (Baron et al., 1999). Additional vocational assessment tools useful for occupational therapists working in vocational placement or transitions tailored to client needs include the Vocational Fit Assessment (worker abilities and job demands) (Persch, Gugiu et al., 2015), the Vocational Index (vocational task independence), the Work Personality Profile (work skills strengths), the Work Readiness Scale (readiness to work), and the Work Task Preference (career preferences) (Mahoney et al., 2021).
- Occupational therapy can contribute to transition teams by intervening to improve functional abilities and health status in postsecondary transition for adults with disabilities through community participation. This has been demonstrated in one particular study, where community

service was significantly related to improved health status and functional abilities (Eismann et al., 2017).

- A study of the vocational interests of women within the criminal justice system generated initial evidence to inform vocational goals which corresponded with the participant's inherent personality characteristics. The O*NET IP vocational interest responses (Holland et al., 1969; National Center for O*NET Development, 2018) and identification of perceived barriers to re-entry employment provided useful client-centered results to inform interventions for transition (Washington et al., 2019).

Summary and Implications: There is a gap in the provision of occupational therapy services in the work transition process (Eismann et al., 2017). This chapter indicates a broad perspective of occupational needs to be explored when designing evidence-informed interventions for vocational/work outcomes (e.g., employment interests and pursuits, seeking and acquisition, and job performance and maintenance) (American Occupational Therapy Association, 2020). Specifically, the Employment Options program for individuals experiencing AIDS revealed the multifaceted challenges that persons with AIDS face, especially health disparities (e.g., unsheltered/homelessness, substance use disorder, mental illness, and cognitive and/or psychomotor impairments), and the importance of considering their narratives to inform tailored work interventions. Of the people with regressive narrative slopes, nearly a third achieved success; however, the mechanisms of impact were unknown and need exploration to determine intervention strategies tailored to narrative slopes. Vocational programming in occupational therapy that address health challenges, physical limitations, environmental factors, and contextual influences on work pursuits are needed for inclusivity of a wide variety of people described in these studies (e.g., postsecondary transition for students with disabilities, women experiencing incarceration).

CLINICAL CASE: COMMUNITY-BASED OCCUPATIONAL THERAPY VOCATIONAL PROGRAMMING DEVELOPMENT AND IMPLEMENTATION

Case History

A team of occupational therapists is developing a community-based program that will offer services for individuals with a record of incarceration (Jaegers et al., 2020). The program will aim to utilize a collaborative approach with community partners to address client physical and behavioral health needs and skills for achieving employment, home management, social network, and leisure goals, among others. Given the supporting evidence in this chapter, consider the following: 1) what key factors should be considered in assessment and interventions, 2) what client factors should be considered to support client goals, and 3) what types of interventions might be most appropriate to address client needs to inform vocational goals and pursuits?

Suggested Answer

Consider the transactional relationship between environment, context, health status, job fit (matching), and personal experiences during the assessment and intervention planning stages. For instance, explore the person's narrative history, personal characteristics, and job interests using the OPHI and O*NET or Vocational Fit Assessment (Persch, Gugiu et al., 2015). Gain an understanding of the person's narrative slope using a trauma-informed approach (e.g., sensitive to the client's trauma experience). Determine how the person interprets life and is motivated to act based on their narrative (Kielhofner et al., 2004) and how their perceptions of work ability match those of their skills and perceived barriers to work (Washington et al., 2019).

Broaden the scope of work interventions to "increase functional abilities and health status" (Eismann et al., 2017, p. 8). For instance, occupational therapy adds value to interventions such as resumé and interview preparation by addressing barriers to work participation, meaningful occupations, and health promotion to support work pursuits. Furthermore, interventions to improve person–environment fit during work performance improve the likelihood of overall job satisfaction (Pfiefer et al., 2018).

References

American Occupational Therapy Association. (2020). Occupational therapy practice framework: Domain and process—Fourth edition. *American Journal of Occupational Therapy,* 74(Supplement_2), Article 7412410010. https://doi.org/10.5014/ajot.2020.74S2001

Baron, K., Kielhofner, G., Goldhammer, V., & Wolenski, J. (1999). *The occupational self assessment (OSA)* [Version 1.0]. Model of Human Occupation Clearinghouse, Department of Occupational Therapy, College of Applied Health Sciences, University of Illinois at Chicago.

Braveman, B., & Helfrich, C. (2001). Occupational identity: Exploring the narratives of three men living with AIDS. *Journal of Occupational Science, 8,* 25–31. https://doi.org/10.1080/14427591.2001.9686486

Eismann, M. M., Weisshaar, R., Capretta, C., Cleary, D. S., Kirby, A. V., & Persch, A. C. (2017). Centennial topics—Characteristics of students receiving occupational therapy services in transition and factors related to postsecondary success. *American*

Journal of Occupational Therapy, 71(3), 7103100010p1–7103100010p8. https://doi.org/10.5014/ajot.2017.024927

Holland, J. L., Whitney, D. R., Cole, N. S., & Richards, J. M. (1969). *An empirical occupational classification derived from a theory of personality and intended for practice and research* (ACT Research Report No. 29). American College Testing Program.

Jaegers, L. A., Skinner, E., Conners, B., Hayes, C., West-Bruce, S., Vaughn, M. G., Smith, D., & Barney, K. F. (2020). Evaluation of the jail-based occupational therapy transition and integration services program for community reentry. *American Journal of Occupational Therapy*, 74, 7403205030. https://doi.org/10.5014/ajot.2020.035287

Kielhofner, G., Braveman, B., Finlayson, M., Paul-Ward, A., Goldbaum, L., & Goldstein, K. (2004). Outcomes of a vocational program for persons with AIDS. *American Journal of Occupational Therapy*, 58(1), 64–72.

Kielhofner, G. (2002). *A model of human occupation: Theory and application* (3rd ed.). Williams & Wilkins.

Kielhofner, G., Mallinson, T., Crawford, C., Nowack, M., Rigby, M., & Henry, A. (1997). *A user's guide to the Occupational Performance History Interview-II (OPHI-II) (Version 2.0)*. Chicago: Model of Human Occupation Clearinghouse, Department of Occupational Therapy, College of Applied Health Sciences, University of Illinois at Chicago.

Mahoney, W. J., Blaskowitz, M. G., & Johnson, K. R. (2021). Occupational therapy–related assessments for adults with intellectual disability: A scoping review. *American Journal of Occupational Therapy*, 75, Article 7503180100. https://doi.org/10.5014/ajot.2021.046342

National Center for O*NET Development. (2018). *About O*NET*. O*NET Resource Center. https://www.onetcenter.org/overview.html

Persch, A. C., Cleary, D. S., Rutkowski, S., Malone, H. C., Darragh, A. R., & Case-Smith, J. D. (2015). Current practices in job matching: A Project SEARCH perspective on transition. *Journal of Vocational Rehabilitation*, 43(3), 259–273. https://doi.org/10.3233/JVR-150774

Persch, A. C., Gugiu, P. C., Onate, J. A., & Cleary, D. S. (2015). Development and psychometric evaluation of the Vocational Fit Assessment (VFA). *American Journal of Occupational Therapy*, 69, 6906180080p1–6906180080p8. http://dx.doi.org/10.5014/ajot.2015.019455

Pfeiffer, B., Brusilovskiy, E., Davidson, A., & Persch, A. (2018). Impact of person-environment fit on job satisfaction for working adults with autism spectrum disorders. *Journal of Vocational Rehabilitation*, 48(1), 49–57.

Velozo, C., Kielhofner, G., & Fisher, G. (1998). *A user's guide to the Worker Role Interview (WRI) (Version 9.0)*. Model of Human Occupation Clearinghouse, Department of Occupational Therapy, College of Applied Health Sciences, University of Illinois at Chicago.

Washington, S. E., Jaegers, L. A., & Katz, I. (2019). Vocational interests of women incarcerated and perceived barriers to societal reentry. *Annals of International Occupational Therapy*, 3(4), 194–199. https://doi.org/10.3928/24761222-20191018-01

19

Impacts of Environmental and Person-Fit Factors on Work Satisfaction and Performance in Adults with Autism Spectrum Disorder (ASD)

ANDREW C. PERSCH

Results of the study identified environmental factors and person-fit as both facilitators and barriers to work satisfaction and performance for adults with ASD. Specifically, adults with ASD identified that social interactions, attitudes, and the physical or sensory environment impacted perceptions of work satisfaction and performance. Person-fit between individual characteristics and job requirements were also identified as an important factor.

PFEIFFER, B., BRAUN, K., KINNEALEY, M., MATCZAKA, M. D., & POLATAJKO, H. (2017). Environmental factors impacting work satisfaction and performance for adults with autism spectrum disorders. *Journal of Vocational Rehabilitation*, 47(1), 1–12.

Original Paper: https://content.iospress.com/articles/journal-of-vocational-rehabilitation/jvr878

Research Question: How do environmental factors impact work satisfaction and performance for adults with ASD?

Funding: American Occupational Therapy Foundation

Year Study Began: 2014

Year Study Published: 2017

Study Location: Urban, university-based

Who Was Studied: Convenience sample of 14 adults (mean age 40, standard deviation = 13.8) with *Diagnostic and Statistical Manual of Mental Disorders,* fourth edition, diagnoses of high-functioning autism, pervasive developmental disorder not otherwise specified, or Asperger's syndrome (hereafter ASD). All participants were English-speaking and employed at least 20 hours a week at the time of the study.

Who Was Excluded: Not applicable.

How Many Participants: 14

Study Overview: Adults with ASD experience poor employment outcomes after high school graduation. This study utilized semi-structured interviews to understand the environmental factors impacting work satisfaction and performance from the perspective of working adults with ASD, a topic not heavily researched. Through open and axial coding of the interview transcripts, the authors identified six major categories of barriers and/or facilitators to work satisfaction and performance (Figure 19.1).

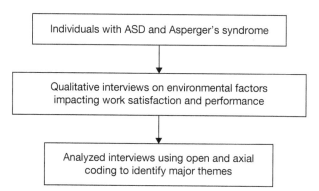

Figure 19.1. Grounded theory study design.

Endpoints: Primary outcome: environmental and person-fit factors that support (+) and/or hinder (−) work satisfaction and performance.

RESULTS

- As shown in Table 19.1, the researchers identified three environmental factors (i.e., social, attitudinal, sensory and physical) and three person-fit factors (i.e., job characteristics, skills and passions, ASD symptoms). Common positive and negative impacts on work satisfaction and performance were found for each of the six factors.
- Environmental factors
  o Social
    - + Social interactions were necessary but challenging. Keeping interactions limited and work-related was preferred.
    - − Small talk was challenging for most. Some expressed discomfort with social interactions at work.
  o Attitudinal
    - + Family support of workers' skills and passions facilitated work satisfaction and performance by providing motivation to work and enhancing job match. A positive self-perception also helped overall attitude at the workplace.
    - − Participants reported negative perceptions and stigmatization from co-workers in the form of patronizing talk and lack of respect as a hindrance to work satisfaction and performance.
  o Sensory and physical
    - + Most participants preferred to work alone in small, clean, and quiet areas. Accommodations/modifications included noise-canceling headphones, dimmable lights, and control over their individual work environment.
    - − Fluorescent lighting, visual distractions, noise level, temperature, and uncomfortable uniforms presented substantial barriers to participants' work satisfaction and performance.
- Person-fit factors
  o Job characteristics
    - + Most participants preferred consistent routines, flexible schedules, short and easy commutes, work benefits, and work autonomy.
    - − Participants reported feeling micromanaged, having limited breaks, and having too few or too many people around as barriers. Other hindrances included long commutes, changes to schedule, and boredom.

o Skills and passions
  • + Participants who found jobs which matched their skills and passions were more satisfied and happier than those who did not.
o ASD symptoms
  • + Consistent schedules and routines helped mitigate symptoms of ASD. Ability to match limited interests and abilities was important to participants.
  • − Participants identified ASD symptoms including social communication, social interactions, anxiety, and sensory issues as barriers to work satisfaction and performance.

Table 19.1. FACTORS THAT SUPPORT AND/OR HINDER WORK SATISFACTION AND PERFORMANCE

Environmental factors	
Social	Interactions and relationships with other co-workers and supervisors in the workplace
Attitudinal	Perceptions of self, co-workers, and workplace environment
Sensory and physical environment	How the physical environment interacts with the participant's senses such as lighting and noise level
Person-fit factors	
Job characteristics	Different job aspects such as the schedule, commute from home, benefits, and breaks during the day
Skills and passions	How well the participant performs the job duties and how meaningful the job is
ASD symptoms	Work-related signs associated with ASD including social impairments, anxiety, sensory processing challenges, and other common symptoms

Criticisms and Limitations: The findings are limited to the perspectives of people with ASD, whereas the thoughts of co-workers, supervisors, and family members are not included in the study. The convenience sample included six male and eight female participants, a proportion that differs from the typical prevalence rate for ASD of approximately four males to one female. The authors note that this qualitative study is not intended for generalization.

Other Relevant Studies and Information:

• Ecological models of human behavior, such as the Occupational Therapy Practice Framework, fourth edition (American Occupational

Therapy Association, 2020), the person–environment–occupation model (Law et al., 1996), and the *International Classification of Functioning* (World Health Organization, 2001), provide a framework for understanding the relationships among the person, environment, and occupation, each of which is useful in considering how to support successful occupational performance in the work context.

- In an extension of the current study, Pfeiffer et al. (2018) found that job satisfaction is increased in adults with ASD when the sensory, social, and relational aspects of the work environment are viewed as more positive.
- The Vocational Fit Assessment (VFA) is a decision-support tool that contains person and environmental factors relevant to postgraduate employment for individuals with intellectual disabilities (e.g., communication skills, work structure, interpersonal skills). The VFA evaluates person–job fit for a range of potential job matches by comparing worker abilities with job demands. These data are used to inform job placement decisions and identify areas of intervention (i.e., skill-building, accommodations, modifications [Persch et al., 2015]).
- In another qualitative study, Hayward et al. (2019) identified that social environmental factors (e.g., co-worker support and understanding) and physical modifications (e.g., sunglasses for light sensitivity) may enable successful employment outcomes.

Summary and Implications: This study demonstrates that adults with ASD experience environmental and person-fit barriers to work satisfaction and performance. Despite these challenges, participants also identified factors that support workplace outcomes and are opportunities for occupational therapy practitioners to intervene with this at-risk population. The study affirms the fundamental tenets of a person–environment–occupation view of human performance.

CLINICAL CASE: OPTIMIZING EMPLOYMENT PERFORMANCE AND SATISFACTION

Case History

An occupational therapist (OT) is working in a vocational rehabilitation setting with a client with ASD who is interested in a position as an information technology call specialist due to the job's alignment with the individual's skill set and knowledge of computer systems. The VFA identified incongruencies in job demands and person characteristics in the areas of interpersonal and communication skills. In addition, the individual has noise sensitivity, and the job demands that the individual works in a shared office space with 10 other individuals. What might the OT recommend to the employer to facilitate a better person–job match? What might the OT recommend to the individual with ASD?

Suggested Answer

Recommendations for the employer could include provision of disability/diversity training for employees, flexibility in implementing accommodation suggestions, identification of potential alternative work spaces, exploration of different desk placements to limit distractions due to noise, and provision of consistency in working hours. Recommendations for the individual with ASD include identifying areas of accommodation (e.g., noise-canceling headphones) and participating in vocational training to develop competency and comfortability in interpersonal communication and self-advocacy. If the employer is unable to make sufficient accommodations to support the individual with ASD, the OT can use the VFA to identify other employment opportunities that align with the individual's interests and skills set.

References

American Occupational Therapy Association. (2020). Occupational therapy practice framework: Domain and process—Fourth edition. *American Journal of Occupational Therapy*, 74(Supplement 2), Article 7412410010.

Hayward, S. M., McVilly, K. R., & Strokes, M. A. (2019). Autism and employment: What works. *Research in Autism Spectrum Disorders*, 60, 48–58.

Law, M., Cooper, B., Strong, S., Stewart, D., Rigby, P., & Letts, L. (1996). The person–environment–occupation model: A transactive approach to occupational performance. *Canadian Journal of Occupational Therapy*, 63(1), 9–23.

Persch, A. C., Gugiu, P. C., Onate, J. A., & Cleary, D. S. (2015). Development and psychometric evaluation of the Vocational Fit Assessment (VFA). *American Journal of Occupational Therapy*, 69, 6906180080p1–6906180080p8. http://dx.doi.org/10.5014/ajot.2015.019455

Pfeiffer, B., Brusilovskiy, E., Davidson, A., & Persch, A. (2018). Impact of person–environment fit on job satisfaction for working adults with autism spectrum disorders. *Journal of Vocational Rehabilitation*, 48(1), 49–57. https://doi.org/10.3233/JVR-170915

World Health Organization. (2001). *International classification of functioning, disability and health: ICF*. https://apps.who.int/iris/handle/10665/42407

SECTION 4

Mental Health

In mental health practice, occupational therapy (OT) practitioners work to support the participation of people across the life span who are labeled with or at risk for mental illness. We do this by understanding a person's occupational history and context, as well as their future aspirations, in a variety of settings (e.g., outpatient clinics, psychiatric hospitals, supported housing, board-and-care homes, and community-based settings). OT practitioners approach practice in mental health with a unique lens, drawing upon our knowledge of occupation, cognition, volition, sensory processing, the impact of the environment, and conceptual models of practice.

In selecting studies for this section, we identified core areas of OT practice in mental health: illness management and recovery, engagement in productive roles, housing, sensory processing, cognition, volition, health and wellness, and substance use. We also sought research in the emerging practice areas of forensic mental health, early intervention for psychosis, and pediatric mental health.

Understanding lived experience is essential to mental health practice in OT. Deegan examines how participants use personal medicine (self-initiated, non-pharmaceutical self-care activities that served to decrease symptoms), while Sutton et al. explore the use of sensory rooms in inpatient psychiatric settings to support individuals' self-regulation. Our commitment to amplify lived experience influenced our decision to invite Tristan Scremin, an "expert by experience,"[1] to co-author the Deegan chapter.

We considered various systematic reviews (e.g., Arbesman & Logsdon, 2011; Arbesman et al., 2013) but opted to omit them because they will continue to be updated based on emerging research. However, we did select the systematic review by Wasmuth et al. as it provides unique insights regarding the value of occupation within recovery from addiction. In searching for evidence of OT's efficacy in mental health, we identified several influential studies which were excluded because they describe interventions not specific to OT practice, such as Substance Abuse and Mental Health Services' Illness Management and Recovery (Hasson-Ohayon et al., 2007), sleep interventions (Faulkner & Bee, 2016), and early intervention for psychosis (McFarlane et al., 2015).

Our final selection of articles addresses sensory processing, lived experience, substance use, health and wellness, supported education, time use, volition, and pediatric mental health. Three articles highlight the value of occupation and OT's role in supporting participation (Deegan, Edgelow & Krupa, and Wasmuth et al.). Gutman et al. and Brown et al. demonstrate OT's value in supported education and wellness. Two studies, Warner et al. and Sutton et al., illustrate the value of sensory processing interventions to reduce distress and improve regulation for people across the life span who may have difficulty participating in top-down, more cognitively oriented interventions.

This section reveals gaps in research on cognition, emerging areas of practice such as forensic mental health, and the full spectrum of care for individuals experiencing housing insecurity. While there are limited high-quality studies when adopting positivist frameworks for evaluating research (e.g., randomized trials), there is a rich body of qualitative research informing mental health practice. Finally, the research represented in this section was conducted by White researchers from the United States, New Zealand, and Canada. While the studies' participants represented diverse populations, most lacked a perspective on equity or acknowledgment of forms of oppression; and there is a need for more participatory approaches that involve experts by experience. We recruited a diverse selection of authors, with both lived and clinical experience, so that perspectives from different racial and cultural groups as well as practice areas were well represented.

Taken as a whole, these articles reflect the importance of supporting participation and recovery through occupation. We feel the chapters in this section

[1] A person with lived experience of mental illness.

provide an orientation to key experiences and interventions that can guide our work as OT practitioners in mental health to support participation.

References

Arbesman, M., Bazyk, S., & Nochajski, S. M. (2013). Systematic review of occupational therapy and mental health promotion, prevention, and intervention for children and youth. *American Journal of Occupational Therapy, 67*, e120–e130. http://dx.doi.org/10.5014/ajot.2013.008359

Arbesman, M., & Logsdon, D. W. (2011). Occupational therapy interventions for employment and education for adults with serious mental illness: A systematic review. *American Journal of Occupational Therapy, 65*(3), 238–246. https://doi.org/10.5014/ajot.2011.001289

Faulkner, S., & Bee, P. (2016). Perspectives on sleep, sleep problems, and their treatment, in people with serious mental illnesses: A systematic review. *PLoS ONE, 11*(9), 1–17. https://doi.org/10.1371/journal.pone.0163486

Hasson-Ohayon, I., Roe, D., & Kravetz, S. (2007). A randomized controlled trial of the effectiveness of the illness management and recovery program. *Psychiatric Services, 58*(11), 1461–1466. https://doi.org/10.1176/ps.2007.58.11.1461

McFarlane, W. R., Levin, B., Travis, L., Lucas, F. L., Lynch, S., Verdi, M., Williams, D., Adelsheim, S., Calkins, R., Carter, C. S., Cornblatt, B., Taylor, S. F., Auther, A. M., McFarland, B., Melton, R., Migliorati, M., Niendam, T., Ragland, J. D., Sale, T., . . . Spring, E. (2015). Clinical and functional outcomes after 2 years in the early detection and intervention for the prevention of psychosis multisite effectiveness trial. *Schizophrenia Bulletin, 41*(1), 30–43. https://doi.org/10.1093/schbul/sbu108

20

Personal Medicine as a Recovery Tool

TRISTAN SCREMIN AND TESSA Z. MILMAN

Personal medicine is evidence of resilience in people with psychiatric disorders. When treatment plans support the personal medicine, resilience, and self assessed health resources of the people who come for help, then clinicians become more effective partners in the journey toward health.

> DEEGAN, P. E. (2005). The importance of personal medicine: A qualitative study of resilience in people with psychiatric disabilities. *Scandinavian Journal of Public Health*, 33(66), 29–35.

Original Paper: https://doi.org/10.1080/14034950510033345

Research Question: How do people with psychiatric disorders "demonstrate the capacity for resilience" (p. 30) within the current treatment climate of over-reliance on pharmaceutical medication?

Funding: State of Kansas and the University of Kansas School of Social Welfare, Lawrence Kansas, USA

Year Study Began: Not available

Year Study Published: 2005

Study Location: Kansas

Who Was Studied: Ten men and 19 women enrolled in a community support program for those labeled with mental health diagnoses. With the exception of three participants, all were using psychiatric medications; 16 had been hospitalized multiple times, and all were currently engaged in community support services; 12 reported a history of substance abuse. The median length of time they had been involved in community support programs was 15 years.

Who Was Excluded: Not available.

How Many Patients: 29

Study Overview: A survey collecting basic demographic information was given to 200 individuals in Kansas who were participating in community support programs designed for individuals labeled with mental illness. From this group, a purposeful sample of 29 individuals was selected in order to ensure diversity of experiences with diagnoses, use of psychiatric medications, race, and residence in urban and rural locations. A few individuals who did not use psychiatric medication were also selected, to provide a diversity of perspectives.

Deegan conducted initial 1-hour interviews with each participant. She disclosed her identity as a person who had used psychiatric medication in her recovery from schizophrenia to help individuals feel comfortable sharing their own experiences. She asked participants to tell "the story of how they came into mental health services and what their experience with psychiatric medication was like" (p. 31). Everyone was asked, "Based on your experience, what is the most important thing that mental health professionals should know in order to be helpful to people using medications?" (p. 31).

The interviews were audiotaped, transcribed, and analyzed using phenomenological methods. To include a participatory component, Deegan reviewed initial results with two focus groups of participants and one additional new participant with a psychiatric disability. These member reflections offered additional perspective about the usefulness, relevance, and accessibility of the findings. She then incorporated the suggestions into the findings.

RESULTS

- In participants' descriptions of their experiences with psychiatric medications, they spontaneously talked about what Deegan termed "personal medicine." This involved engaging in activities to find meaning and purpose in their lives and to take care of themselves. The range of activities was varied but included parenting, going for walks, taking time off, calling a friend, and working.

- Participants explained that engaging in this personal medicine decreased their positive and negative symptoms and reduced hospitalizations, increased wellness, and improved their coping. Despite the value of these activities, they did not share their personal medicine with providers, often because they felt that the providers might not approve. Sometimes personal medicine involved doing activities that they felt their providers would discourage such as using drugs or alcohol or having sex. Others might have been willing to share their experience of personal medicine with providers, but they were never asked about it.

- When taking psychotropic medication interfered with individuals' abilities to engage in their valued occupations or personal medicine, they often stopped taking medication as prescribed. For example, one woman described stopping her psychotropic medication because it interfered with her desire to take care of her children, which resulted in increased symptoms and decreased quality of life.

- The study findings illustrate how incorporating personal medicine into treatment can support recovery. Deegan advocates for individuals to craft a power statement, which can help the person declare how their personal medicine must be considered as an integral part of their recovery.

Personal medicine

- Is self-initiated
- Leads to reduced symptoms
- Helps people avoid undesirable outcomes such as hospitalization
- Improves mood, thoughts, behaviors, and overall sense of well-being
- May not be traditionally conceived as health-promoting, for example, using drugs
- Is often not disclosed to providers
- Is sometimes disrupted by psychiatric medication

Two main categories of personal medicine were identified:

- Activities that give meaning and purpose to life
- Specific self-care strategies

Criticisms and Limitations: Individuals were only interviewed once. Additional time and interviews, possibly combined with participant observation, may have led to richer data and findings. The first author conducted the study because of her concern about over prescription of psychiatric medication; this may have influenced the way she conducted interviews and analyzed the data, potentially overemphasizing participants' reported use of non-pharmaceutical strategies.

Other Relevant Studies and Information: Some studies confirm Deegan's findings regarding how individuals labeled with mental illness use occupations in recovery. Lal et al. (2013) explored how young people with psychosis experienced well-being through engaging in activities they valued. Others complicate her findings. For example, Milbourn et al. (2015) explored how individuals labeled with mental illness often felt trapped and bored by a routine of occupations structured around receiving care from others and financial management.

Other studies provide guidance for practitioners to support individuals in using personal medicine and/or occupations in recovery. Programs specifically incorporating occupation into recovery with positive outcomes include Action over Inertia (Edgelow & Krupa, 2011), Common Ground Intervention (Macdonald-Wilson et al., 2013), and Behavioral Activation for Negative Symptoms (Mairs et al., 2011).

Summary and Implications: This study demonstrates that resilience is built in many ways, including through personal medicine, which occupational therapists (OTs) often describe as meaningful occupations. Personal medicine is often overlooked by providers focusing on deficit-based approaches, yet engaging in these personal wellness strategies was a key factor for recovery for many of the participants. Providers can build trust and support recovery by asking about and supporting individuals in using personal medicine.

CLINICAL CASE: MY NICOTINE ALARM

Case History

Alex's (he/him) psychiatrist at an outpatient mental health clinic has referred him to the OT to help him quit smoking. He currently smokes 20 cigarettes a day. When the OT spoke with Alex about quitting, he explained that smoking is the way that he relaxes himself and that it helps him connect with others when he sits outside, taking a break. Alex identifies as gay and Latinx and shares that sitting outside with other smokers has helped him become part of a queer community. He also shares that smoking has helped him stay out of the hospital. Alex explains that smoking provides a kind of "nicotine alarm," cueing him to change his environment and take frequent 5-minute breaks and do deep breathing for 5 minutes, which he feels helps him manage his symptoms. What should the OT recommend to the psychiatrist in the next team meeting when they are talking about Alex?

Suggested Answer

In the team meeting, it will be important for the OT to convey that while smoking is detrimental to health, it is Alex's "personal medicine" and that Alex perceives that it helps improve his quality of life by helping him take breaks and change his environment when stressed. Trying to get him to stop smoking immediately may hinder Alex's trust and disrupt his recovery. Deegan writes that "Clinicians should routinely inquire about personal medicine and what patients are already doing to help themselves with their distress" (p. 35). It will be important to ask about Alex's use of cigarettes as personal medicine and, if he expresses the desire to quit smoking, to help him identify and use other types of personal medicine that could potentially replace smoking.

References

Edgelow, M., & Krupa, T. (2011). Randomized controlled pilot study of an occupational time-use intervention for people with serious mental illness. *American Journal of Occupational Therapy, 65*, 267–276. https://doi.org/10.5014/ajot.2011.001313

Lal, S., Ungar, M., Leggo, C. Malla, A., Frankish, J., & Suto, M. J. (2013). Well-being and engagement in valued activities: Experiences of young people with psychosis. *OTJR: Occupation, Participation and Health, 33*(4), 190–197. https://doi.org/10.3928/15394492-20130912-02

MacDonald-Wilson, K. L., Deegan, P. E., Hutchison, S. L., Parrotta, N., & Schuster, J. M. (2013). Integrating personal medicine into service delivery: Empowering people in recovery. *Psychiatric Rehabilitation Journal, 36*(4), 258–263. https://doi.org/10.1037/prj0000027

Mairs, H., Lovell, K., Campbell, M., & Keeley, P. (2011). Development and pilot investigation of behavioral activation for negative symptoms. *Behavior Modification, 35*(5), 486–506. https://doi.org/10.1177/0145445511411706

Milbourn, B., McNamara, B., & Buchanan, A. (2015). The lived experience of everyday activity for individuals with severe mental illness. *Health Sociology Review, 24*(3), 270–282. https://doi.org/10.1080/14461242.2015.1034747

Occupational Time-Use Intervention for People with Serious Mental Illness

Action over Inertia

CAROL LAMBDIN-PATTAVINA

Action over Inertia

> The results of this pilot study provide evidence that the [Action over Inertia] intervention can be effective in influencing occupational balance.
>
> EDGELOW, M., & KRUPA, T. (2011). Randomized controlled pilot study of an occupational time-use intervention for people with serious mental illness. *American Journal of Occupational Therapy, 65*(3), 267–276.

Original Paper: https://pubmed.ncbi.nlm.nih.gov/21675332/

Research Question: Does participation in a 12-week Action over Inertia (AOI) intervention improve occupational balance and engagement among community-dwelling adults living with severe and persistent mental illness?

Funding: Not available

Year Study Began: 2007

Year Study Published: 2011

Study Location: Ontario, Canada (cities included Belleville, Kingston, and Ottawa)

Who Was Studied: Community-dwelling adults living with severe mental illness (SMI) who received treatment delivered by a local Assertive Community Treatment (ACT) team.

Who Was Excluded: Not available

How Many Patients: 24

Study Overview: See Figure 21.1.

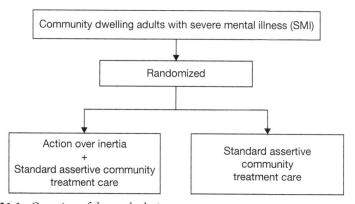

Figure 21.1. Overview of the study design.

Study Intervention: Subjects in the intervention group participated in a 12-week AOI program in addition to the standard care they received via ACT teams located in various urban areas. The control group continued to receive ACT services as usual. Intervention group participants met with the study occupational therapists in weekly one-on-one sessions to complete the AOI program over the 12-week period.

The AOI program posits that limited occupational engagement is a public health issue related to the fear and stigma that continue to shroud mental illness and limit opportunities for activity participation. The Canadian Model of Occupational Performance and the Recovery Model served as theoretical frameworks upon which the AOI program was developed. These models place the individual at the center of their journey toward greater health and wellness and rely heavily on creating a therapeutic environment that supports growth, empowerment, and self-advocacy.

Interventions used in the AOI program include psychoeducation and a variety of cognitive and behavioral strategies to facilitate action. The program is manualized, and the workbook includes interventions that target the following five topical areas: assessing the need for change and eliciting interest in the change process, reflecting upon current patterns of occupational engagement, education regarding the relationship between SMI and patterns of occupational engagement, goal-setting, and ongoing assessment of goals and progress.

Follow-Up: Researchers tested all study participants at baseline and at the end of the 12-week intervention via time-use diaries and the Profiles of Occupational Engagement for People with Schizophrenia (POES).

Endpoints:

- Patterns of time use which result in occupational balance/imbalance (24-hour time-use diaries)
- Occupational engagement (POES)
- Clinical utility of the AOI program (post-intervention questionnaires)

RESULTS

- Twenty-four participants were randomized into an intervention group ($n = 14$) and a control group ($n = 10$), and 18 completed the study (intervention group $n = 10$ and control group $n = 8$) (Table 21.1).
- While the intervention group was 1) older and 2) diagnosed with an SMI longer than the control group, researchers statistically analyzed the influence of these factors on outcomes; and the results yielded no significant impact.
- Differences in occupational balance between the intervention and control groups were statistically significant for sleep. The intervention group slept 47 minutes less each night on average post-intervention versus the control group that slept an average of 22 minutes more each night following the 12-week study period. The effect size for the sleep difference between the intervention and control groups was large and calculated at $d = 0.86$.
- The intervention group used the additional time they gained from sleeping less to engage in general activities rather than participating in

non-health-promoting behaviors, and no activity-specific time-use trends emerged.

- No statistically significant differences between the intervention and control groups were found on the POES.
- With regard to clinical utility, participants responded positively to the questionnaire following the AOI program, and many noted that they experienced increased time-use awareness and improved feelings of well-being as a result of intervention participation. The occupational therapists who administered the study program responded positively to the program's content, structure, and flexibility, although some wanted greater autonomy to alter the program timeline based on clients' needs and preferences.

Table 21.1. DEMOGRAPHICS

Demographics

Characteristic	CONTROL GROUP ($n = 8$) Mean	TREATMENT GROUP ($n = 10$) Mean	p
Age	32.38	44.60	.016
Years since diagnosis	10.75	21.20	.026

Occupational Balance

Time Use Category (Hours)	CONTROL GROUP ($n = 8$) Mean	TREATMENT GROUP ($n = 10$) Mean	p
Sleep			
Pretest	10.75	10.88	.89
Change at Posttest	0.37	−0.78	.05

Criticisms and Limitations: Noted limitations included small sample size ($n = 18$) limiting generalizability, sample uniformity (all participants were service users of ACT programs), and attrition (four intervention participants left the study, potentially leaving behind those who responded more positively, which might have skewed results). Additionally, no sensitivity data exist on the POES, and the instrument may not have detected statistically significant changes in such a small sample size. Finally, maintenance of intervention gains is unknown as no follow-up measures were used.

Other Relevant Studies and Information:

- The link between occupation and health has been theoretically made (Wilcock, 2007), and new research is supporting this theory with evidence (Newport & Clarke, 2020).
- Diverse individuals living with SMI tend to be occupationally disengaged for both internal reasons (manifestations of the illness) and external reasons (social exclusion and stigma), which can lead to intensification of the mental illness as well as physical health concerns (Pooremamali et al., 2017).
- The mortality gap between those living with SMI and their cohort who do not have SMI is wide. High rates of heart disease, diabetes, and respiratory disease contribute to this gap and have been linked to types and degree of occupational engagement (Erlangsen et al., 2017).
- When used in a group setting, AOI facilitated participants' ability to make change and understand the relationship between health and time use as well as leaders' ability to facilitate change for improved health outcomes (Rees et al., 2021).

Summary and Implications: Occupation is understood to enhance health and well-being, but few studies have been conducted to demonstrate the impact of interventions on occupational engagement and balance with individuals experiencing SMI. Statistically significant differences in time spent in sleep between the intervention and control groups along with positive qualitative feedback from the study can be used to frame thinking about time use and occupational balance. The AOI study provides promising outcomes and a clear path for expansion and replication of the study with other mental health populations and settings. AOI's emphasis on occupational engagement as a public health issue is in concert with occupational therapy's understanding that people living with SMI are inextricably embedded in and influenced by their contexts and environments; failure to acknowledge and address these broader contexts and environments will result in historically poorer outcomes for this population.

CLINICAL CASE: AOI IN ACTION

Case History

Gerardo (he/him), a 50-year-old Latinx male client, currently resides in community-based supportive housing. He experienced insecure attachments in childhood and entered foster care at the age of 6. He was diagnosed with bipolar disorder at the age of 14 and schizoaffective disorder at the age of 22. An inconsistent work history, low socioeconomic status, and decreased social support left this client isolated with few resources; and his use of alcohol and cigarette smoking has steadily increased in recent years. Gerardo is currently unemployed and was recently diagnosed with mild chronic obstructive pulmonary disease. He typically sleeps 12+ hours/night and spends waking hours watching TV, smoking, drinking if finances permit, and occasionally sitting outside where he greets others who live in the same housing complex. Two times per week, he attends a social program for several hours but lately has not attended consistently due to increased breathing difficulty and difficulty taking action.

What outcomes of the AOI study relate directly to this case? What information related to this client's history and current functioning would indicate use of the AOI program?

Suggested Answer

Gerardo is sleeping 12+ hours per night, which has been linked to increased risk for mortality (Hossin, 2016) and health conditions such as coronary artery disease (Yang et al., 2015). Results of the AOI study indicate that this manualized program, which uses psychoeducational, cognitive, and behavioral strategies, can be useful in decreasing the amount of time this client spends engaged in sleep. An occupational therapy practitioner using the AOI program could assist Gerardo in identifying where and how he spends his time to then assess whether or not that time-use configuration supports or hinders overall health and wellness. Through education and use of cognitive and behavioral strategies, the client may be able to make notable shifts in time usage. The time that he may recover secondary to decreased time spent sleeping can be used to engage in other meaningful activities that he identifies in the context of completing the program. Aside from potential outcomes related to increased awareness of time use and improved life satisfaction as noted by study participants, decreased sleep may lead to improved physical health outcomes such as lowered risk of heart disease.

References

Erlangsen, A., Andersen, P. K., Toender, A., Laursen, T. M., Nordentoft, M., & Canudas-Romo, V. (2017). Cause-specific life-years lost in people with mental disorders: A nationwide, register-based cohort study. *The Lancet Psychiatry*, 4(12), 937–945. https://pubmed.ncbi.nlm.nih.gov/29122573/

Hossin, M. Z. (2016). From habitual sleep hours to morbidity and mortality: Existing evidence, potential mechanisms, and future agenda. *Sleep Health*, 2(2), 146–153. https://pubmed.ncbi.nlm.nih.gov/28923258/

Newport, A., & Clarke, C. (2020). The experiences of people with severe mental health conditions participating in the Occupation Matters Programme: An interpretative phenomenological analysis. *British Journal of Occupational Therapy, 83*(10), 620–630. https://journals.sagepub.com/doi/full/10.1177/0308022619899014

Pooremamali, P., Morville, A.-L., & Eklund, M. (2017). Barriers to continuity in the pathway toward occupational engagement among ethnic minorities with mental illness. *Scandinavian Journal of Occupational Therapy, 24*(4), 259–268. https://pubmed. ncbi.nlm.nih.gov/27402119/

Rees, E. F., Ennals, P., & Fossey, E. (2021). Implementing an Action over Inertia group program in community residential rehabilitation services: Group participant and facilitator perspectives. *Frontiers in Psychiatry, 12,* Article 624803. https://pubmed.ncbi. nlm.nih.gov/33603690/

Wilcock, A. A. (2007). Occupation and health: Are they one and the same? *Journal of Occupational Science, 14*(1), 3–8. https://www.tandfonline.com/doi/abs/10.1080/ 14427591.2007.9686577?cookieSet=1

Yang, X., Chen, H., Li, S., Pan, L., & Jia, C. (2015). Association of sleep duration with the morbidity and mortality of coronary artery disease: A meta-analysis of prospective studies. *Heart, Lung & Circulation, 24*(12), 1180–1190. https://www.sciencedir ect.com/science/article/pii/S1443950615013566

22

Optimizing Arousal to Manage Aggression

ERIN MCINTYRE

Narrative analysis of interview and focus group data [suggests] that modifications to the environment and the use of soothing stimuli moderate or optimize arousal and promote an ability to adaptively regulate emotion.

SUTTON, D., WILSON, M., VAN KESSEL, K., & VANDERPYL, J. (2013).
Optimizing arousal to manage aggression:
A pilot study of sensory modulation. *International Journal of Mental Health Nursing, 22,* 500–511.

Original Paper: https://doi.org/10.1111/inm.12010

Research Question: Does the use of sensory modulation strategies in inpatient psychiatric settings improve the range of effective options within aggression management practices, resulting in reduced seclusion and restraint?

Funding: None.

Year Study Began: 2009

Year Study Published: 2013

Study Location: New Zealand

Who Was Studied:

- 40 clinical staff across four inpatient mental health units
- 20 service users (patients) across four inpatient mental health units

Who Was Excluded: Not applicable

How Many Patients: 20

Study Overview: This study examined the impact of sensory-based approaches (i.e., a sensory room) in inpatient mental health settings as a means to moderate arousal and facilitate emotional regulation of service users. The study examines differences in service users' responses to sensory inputs, informed by recent theoretical advances in the neurophysiology of emotional regulation and polyvagal theory (DeWall et al., 2011; Porges, 2001). The study evaluates the use of a bottom-up sensory approach as a means for de-escalation and prevention of aggression, in contrast to the purely cognitive focus of the General Aggression Model, which has been utilized historically as a key framework for understanding aggression.

An inductive, qualitative approach using focus groups and interviews was conducted in two phases to evaluate the sensory modulation intervention (sensory room). In both phases, a semi-structured interview was used with the clinical staff from the units and service users who had been discharged from the units, in which they described their experiences using the intervention. All interviews and focus groups were conducted by a member of the research team who was not employed by the mental health service.

Study Intervention: A sensory modulation intervention was piloted in four inpatient mental health units (three adult units, one youth unit), in the form of a sensory room. Clinical staff received training in the theory and principles of sensory modulation and were introduced to the sensory equipment to be used in the room, which included items such as a massage chair, a rocking chair, a beanbag, weighted blankets, "stress" balls, audio of relaxing sounds, aromatic oils, and adjustable ambient lighting, among others. Service users were oriented to the sensory room as part of the admission process. When service users' distress escalated, access to the sensory room was facilitated by a member of staff. Staff were also encouraged to offer use of the sensory room at the earliest signs of escalation.

In the sensory room itself, staff supported the service user to explore sensory equipment to support self-regulation.

Follow-Up: The research was conducted in two phases. The first phase occurred in 2009 and focused on initial experiences of the implementation of the sensory modulation rooms. The second phase occurred in 2011 and focused on how the intervention had evolved in the four units.

RESULTS

The qualitative findings indicate that use of sensory modulation interventions facilitated de-escalation of arousal or regulation of emotion and increased interpersonal connections and self-management of arousal in the majority of those who utilized them. Three main themes representing the experiences of service users and staff using the sensory room emerged from the analysis:

- *Facilitating a calm state*—Use of the sensory room reduced arousal and "facilitated a calm state" (Sutton et al., p. 503).
- *Enhancing interpersonal connection*—Sensory modulation facilitated the development of trust and rapport between staff and service users. The service user perspective indicated that the presence of staff in a supportive role in the sensory room was at times as important as the sensory equipment itself (Sutton et al., p. 505).
- *Supporting self-management*—Use of the sensory room and equipment facilitated self-awareness among service users and allowed for a shared understanding about sensory preferences between service users and staff. Staff and service users also commented on the importance of using the sensory strategies upon discharge, as a means to support self-management and recovery longer term (Sutton et al., p. 506).

Subthemes:

- *Soothing and grounding effect*—Participants experienced a grounding effect from somatic sensation and felt soothed by the equipment in the sensory room.
- *Shifting of attention and affect*—Drawing attention to sensations in the body or elements of the environment allowed for distraction from distressing experiences.

- *Increased sense of control*—An increased sense of control was facilitated through use of sensory tools, which helped to mitigate the distressing effect of institutional barriers and distressing symptoms.
- *Expression and release*—This was achieved through the use of sensory equipment which allowed for participants to feel regulated enough to open up emotionally to staff or to release pent-up energy.

Criticisms and Limitations: Although one of the inpatient units included in the study was for youth, no young people participated in focus groups or interviews after discharge. There was also no control group utilized.

Member checking or member reflections by getting participants' feedback on the findings could help deepen the understanding of experiences.

An observational component to the study could capture additional dimensions of the experience of using the sensory room.

Because this study was qualitative in design, it elicited information primarily related to the meaningfulness and relevance of the intervention; therefore, additional research is needed to examine the intervention's effectiveness. To do so, future research should assess the intervention with the use of a validated tool for identifying the likelihood of potential aggression and/or an objective measure of autonomic arousal, which could demonstrate how sensory interventions utilize the ventral vagus to optimize arousal, resulting in more effective management of aggression.

Other Relevant Studies and Information:

- A scoping review (Scanlan & Novak, 2015) found that sensory interventions were effective in reducing distress and supporting client self-management. It was noted that sensory interventions should be combined with other approaches that target changing the organizational culture in order to be effective in reducing seclusion and restraint.
- In response to the Substance Abuse and Mental Health Services Administration's (2010) national initiative Promoting Alternatives to Seclusion and Restraint, to reduce the use of seclusion and restraint in inpatient mental health settings, Champagne and Stromberg (2004) argue that using sensory approaches provides an important mechanism for delivering trauma-informed approaches to support consumers' self-regulation, as well as promote recovery.

- Another pilot study (Novak et al., 2012) that studied the use of a sensory room in an inpatient mental health setting found the sensory room to be effective in reducing distress. The use of weighted blankets was found to be particularly effective.

Summary and Implications: The results of the study support the development of theory and practice related to the prevention, reduction, and management of aggression. The inclusion of sensory modulation interventions in inpatient mental health settings plays an important role in optimizing arousal and promoting emotional regulation. Sensory interventions provide a bottom-up approach to facilitate self-management of distress when an individual's affective state makes it difficult to employ cognitive strategies alone. Sensory interventions have the potential to lead to decreased rates of seclusion and restraint, as well as improve service users' self-management of distressing symptoms.

CLINICAL CASE: SENSORY STRATEGIES FOR SELF-REGULATION IN INPATIENT PSYCHIATRIC SETTINGS

Case History

Felicia (she/her), a 46-year-old female, is admitted to an inpatient psychiatric unit after an exacerbation of symptoms related to a diagnosis of schizophrenia that has left her afraid to leave her apartment and to eat anything other than cans of fruit and unable to sleep for several weeks. She has been unable to care for herself safely as a result and has been staying awake at night for the past 2 weeks due to her paranoia and fear for her safety. Felicia's neighbors became concerned after not seeing her for weeks and asked that a wellness check be carried out. Once admitted to the inpatient unit, she appears to be easily startled by loud noises, is seen pacing the hallways, and becomes increasingly irritable. What intervention strategies might the occupational therapist consider utilizing to address the heightened levels of distress the patient is exhibiting?

Suggested Answer

Given Felicia's apparent arousal level and distress, she should be invited to utilize the sensory room with a member of staff to facilitate emotional regulation and promote a calm and relaxed state, as soon as possible. Utilizing the sensory room will allow the client to have control over the noise level and access to sensory modalities that promote relaxation, such as weighted blankets and a rocking chair. According to Sutton et al., these sensory modalities may help the client to shift her attention away from distressing symptoms to focus on somatic sensations in the body. With regular use of the sensory room, Felicia may experience a decrease in arousal, which could facilitate better quality of sleep and prevent an escalation of distress and irritability. Use of the sensory room may also be helpful in facilitating the development of trust and rapport with staff, of whom she may be suspicious.

References

Champagne, T., & Stromberg, N. (2004). Sensory approaches in inpatient psychiatric settings: Innovative alternatives to seclusion and restraint. *Journal of Psychosocial Nursing and Mental Health Services, 42*(9), 34–44. https://doi.org/10.3928/02793695-20040901-06

DeWall, C. N., Anderson, C. A., & Bushman, B. (2011). The general aggression model: Theoretical extensions to violence. *Psychology of Violence, 1,* 245–258. https://doi.org/10.1037/A0023842

Novak, T., Scanlan, J., McCaul, D., MacDonald, N., & Clarke, T. (2012). Pilot study of a sensory room in an acute inpatient psychiatric unit. *Australasian Psychiatry, 20*(5), 401–406. https://doi.org/10.1177/1039856212459585

Porges, S. W. (2001). The polyvagal theory: Phylogenetic substrates of a social nervous system. *International Journal of Psychophysiology, 42,* 123–146. https://doi.org/10.1016/s0167-8760(01)00162-3

Scanlan, J., & Novak, T. (2015). Sensory approaches in mental health: A scoping review. *Australian Occupational Therapy Journal, 62*(5), 277–285. https://doi.org/10.1111/1440-1630.12224

Substance Abuse and Mental Health Services Administration. (2010). *Promoting alternatives to the use of seclusion and restraint: A national strategy to prevent seclusion and restraint in behavioral health services*(Issue brief No. 1). US Department of Health and Human Services.

23

Somatically Based Regulation Intervention for Adolescents Who Have Experienced Complex Trauma

JESSICA DE BRUN

This pilot, quasi-experimental outcome study provides preliminary support for potential effectiveness of the SMART [Somatic Motor Arousal Regulation Treatment] intervention model in reducing internalizing symptoms associated with complex trauma in youth.

WARNER, E., SPINAZZOLA, J., WESTCOTT, A., GUNN, C., & HODGDON, H. (2014). The body can change the score: Empirical support of somatic regulation in the treatment of traumatized adolescents. The Journal of Child and Adolescent Trauma, 7(4), 237–246.

Original Paper: https://doi.org/10.1007/s40653-014-0030-z

Research Question: Does the contribution of somatic regulation intervention stabilize skill-building in complex trauma treatment for adolescents?

Funding: Not applicable

Year Study Began: Not available

Year Study Published: 2014

Study Location: Two residential treatment centers located across the northeastern United States

Who Was Studied: Adolescents with histories of complex trauma in residential care ranging in age from 13 to 20 years.

- 10% male, 90% female
- 55% Caucasian, 20% Hispanic/Latino, 16% African American, 7% biracial
- 48% had three or more comorbid diagnoses, 42% two diagnoses, 10% one diagnosis
- 77% had experienced emotional abuse, 74% neglect, 73% impaired caregiving, 70% physical abuse, 55% sexual abuse

Who Was Excluded: Adolescents with a history of complex trauma in two residential care facilities were assigned to either the treatment as usual (TAU) group or the SMART group. Adolescents in the SMART group were selected based on their therapists' perception of clinical need related to difficulty talking in sessions, problems with affect, and daily behavioral dysregulation. SMART group participants were matched to TAU participants by age, ethnicity, number and types of trauma exposure, and symptoms.

How Many Patients: 31

Study Overview: This quasi-experimental matched control design compared once-a-week SMART intervention versus TAU (Figure 23.1).

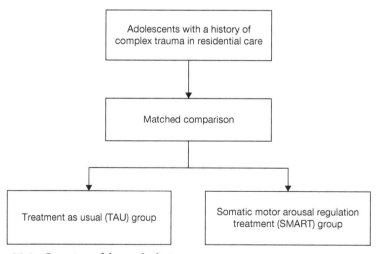

Figure 23.1. Overview of the study design.

Study Intervention: Participants in the TAU group participated in weekly individualized psychotherapy sessions. These sessions occurred in various traditional, office-based talk therapy milieus that were already part of the youths' routine and environmental context.

Participants in the SMART group were invited to explore the SMART intervention room. The SMART intervention room was developed based on the SMART intervention manual and adapted for an adolescent residential population. The therapeutic space offered opportunities to experiment with and explore sensory integration and sensory-motor equipment such as fitness balls, large crash pillows, a mini-trampoline, and a balance beam. Therapists were trained in co-regulation techniques and in identifying and tracking the type of body movement and sensory-motor input sought by the adolescents. With this knowledge the therapists were able to aid in the adolescent's awareness of how to self- (or co-) regulate. Treatment duration was determined on an individual clinical basis by clinicians and supervisors. An invitational approach was utilized and determined most effective for this population.

Follow-Up: Participants were assessed at baseline and at a median of 9 months after initiating treatment.

Endpoints: The study's primary outcomes were as follows:

- Internalizing and externalizing symptoms as measured by the Child Behavior Checklist (CBCL), including subscales assessing somatic complaints and anxious/depressed symptoms.
- Trauma symptom severity as measured by the Posttraumatic Stress Disorder Reaction Index (PTSD-RI), including subscales assessing avoidance and overarousal.

RESULTS

The study findings demonstrate the effectiveness of the SMART model intervention in reducing symptoms such as anxious and depressed mood in adolescents with a history of complex trauma. In addition, the study identified improvement of somatic regulation and hyperarousal symptoms related to PTSD.

- The CBCL Internalizing scale demonstrated a significant reduction of symptoms for the SMART group ($F = 7.286, p = 0.011$) when compared to the TAU group.
- Secondary analysis of the CBCL Internalizing subscale indicated a significant improvement on the CBCL Somatic Complaints ($F = 6.523,$

$p = 0.016$) and Anxious/Depressed ($F = 5.555$, $p = 0.025$) subscales from pre- to post-treatment for the SMART group.
- Reduction of symptoms demonstrated on both the CBCL Externalizing scale and the PTSD-RI indicated no significant difference between the SMART and TAU groups.
- A trend for lower PTSD-RI Overarousal subscale scores ($p = 0.06$) was observed for the SMART group compared with the TAU group.
- While reductions were noted on the PTSD-RI Re-experiencing subscale, no statistically significant differences were identified for the SMART and TAU groups.
- Both the SMART and TAU groups reported lower PTSD-RI Avoidance subscale scores at post-treatment, but no statistically significant changes were found within or across groups (see Table 23.1).

Table 23.1. CHANGES IN TRAUMA SYMPTOMS FROM PRE- TO POST-TREATMENT BY GROUP

Group (n)	CBCL Internalizing		CBCL Externalizing		PTSD-RI Overall	
	Pre	Post	Pre	Post	Pre	Post
SMART (10)	64.9 (5.0)	58.7 (6.5)	65.3 (4.1)	63.3 (3.8)	36.6 (11.1)	29.8 (11.4)
TAU (21)	61.6 (7.7)	63.7 (6.1)	62.5 (7.2)	59.8 (8.9)	29.6 (13.5)	29.7 (11.6)

Values are mean (standard deviation).

Criticisms and Limitations: Assignment to the SMART and TAU groups was not random; therefore, results may be due to underlying differences between groups (i.e., confounding factors). The study utilized videotape to address fidelity; however, some youth were not permitted to be videotaped, leading to the preclusion of some SMART group participants, which potentially skewed the study sample. The small sample size limits the ability to examine differences among types of trauma within groups. Additionally, the SMART model was designed in collaboration with occupational therapists and is within the scope of occupational therapy practice; however, the self- and co-regulation of participants in the SMART model group were monitored by clinicians who were psychotherapists.

Other Relevant Studies and Information:

- For youth in the juvenile justice system, occupational therapy is well positioned to address dysregulation of the sympathetic and parasympathetic nervous systems impacted by chronic childhood trauma through sensory interventions such as sensory diets, comfort/ sensory rooms, environmental modifications, and meaningful activities (Dowdy et al., 2020).

- The Trauma Resiliency Model emphasizes the neuroscientific theory of somatic awareness as a "bottom-up" approach to trauma informed care, highlighting the importance of sensory approaches as an initial step to therapy (Grabbe & Miller-Karas, 2018).
- The SAFE PLACE program, a multidisciplinary intervention program, was found to be suitable and safe for children with complex trauma and sensory processing disorder, with high caregiver satisfaction (May-Benson & Teasdale, 2019).

Summary and Implications: For adolescents who have experienced complex trauma and exhibit developmental disruption in self-regulation or who have the inability to utilize language-based psychotherapy, the SMART treatment model may be a beneficial occupational therapy intervention for decreasing symptoms of behavioral dysregulation Additionally, the SMART model utilizes sensory integration and sensory-motor strategies, which are useful for occupational therapists addressing sensory processing disorder and self- and co-regulation concerns impacting functional occupational engagement.

CLINICAL CASE: APPLICATION OF SOMATIC SENSORY INTERVENTION FOR YOUTH WHO HAVE EXPERIENCED COMPLEX TRAUMA

Case History

Anthony (he/him) is a 15-year-old male who came to the residential treatment center after placement in multiple foster homes, most recently with his maternal grandmother. The Department of Children and Family Services removed Anthony from his maternal grandmother's care after an inpatient psychiatric hospital stay due to an immediate risk of harming his grandmother. Anthony had initially been placed in his grandmother's care at 8 years old, after his father and mother were incarcerated for the non-premeditated killing of Anthony's maternal grandfather. It is believed that Anthony witnessed the killing.

Anthony has not been successful in language-based psychotherapy and is being referred to the occupational therapist for help with regulating his anxious behaviors, agitation, and rapid breathing during psychotherapy. What intervention strategies might the occupational therapist consider while addressing self-regulation during psychotherapy?

Suggested Answer

The client's behaviors illustrated in the vignette are typical of youth who have experienced significant complex developmental trauma. The treating occupational therapists should employ somatically based sensory-motor arousal regulation techniques such as those defined in the SMART treatment model described in the study. In addition, this study found that the client should be invited to experiment and explore various sensory-motor strategies rather than prearranged ones. This invitation method promotes the therapeutic relationship and increases the probability of youth engaging in sensory-motor strategies routinely. Furthermore, the therapist should consider observing the client and noticing when regulatory tools might be initiated as an opportunity for co-regulation and successful sensory-motor regulation exploration.

References

Dowdy, R., Estes, J., Linkugel, M., & Dvornak, M. (2020). Trauma, sensory processing, and the impact of occupational therapy on youth behavior in juvenile corrections. *Occupational Therapy in Mental Health*, 36(4), 373–393. https://doi.org/10.1080/0164212X.2020.1823930

Grabbe, L., & Miller-Karas, E. (2018). The trauma resiliency model: A "bottom-up" intervention for trauma psychotherapy. *Journal of the American Psychiatric Nurses Association*, 24(1), 76–84. https://doi.org/10.1177/1078390317745133

May-Benson, T. A., & Teasdale, A. (2019). Safe place: Clinical utility and feasibility of a multidisciplinary intervention for children with sensory processing disorder and complex trauma—A feasibility study. *Journal of Adolescent Trauma*, 13(2), 207–216. https://doi.org/10.1007/s40653-019-00281-1

Supported Education for Adults with Psychiatric Disabilities

RASHELLE NAGATA

The results support the effectiveness of the Bridge Program and suggest that the program helped participants to increase their skill level in basic academic areas, improve professional behaviors and social skills needed for school and work settings, and gain the confidence to test their skills in the larger community.

GUTMAN, S., KERNER, R., ZOMBEK, I., DULEK, J., & RAMSEY, C. (2009). Supported education for adults with psychiatric disabilities: Effectiveness of an occupational therapy program. *American Journal of Occupational Therapy, 63,* 245–254.

Original Paper: https://ajot.aota.org/article.aspx?articleid=1865836

Research Question: Is a supported education program for adults with psychiatric disabilities effective in promoting higher education enrollment or employment?

Funding: None

Year Study Began: 2006

Year Study Published: 2009

Study Location: New York, NY

Who Was Studied: Adults (aged 19–55) with a psychiatric disability:

- 58% male, 42% female
- 39% Hispanic, 37% African American, 21% White
- Diagnoses: 42% schizophrenia, 29% schizoaffective disorder, 16% bipolar disorder, 13% depression
- Approximately 56% previously hospitalized due to psychiatric illness

Participant eligibility was determined by performance in most daily living activities, interest in further education, and basic reading and writing skills.

Who Was Excluded: Participants were excluded if not fluent in English or diagnosed with an active substance abuse disorder.

How Many Patients: 38

Study Overview: This study used a randomized controlled trial design to measure the effectiveness of a supported education program—the Bridge Program—in supporting adults with psychiatric disabilities who wish to pursue education and vocational training. Study participants were randomized to either the control group, who received mental health treatment as usual, or the experimental group, who attended the Bridge Program in addition to their treatment as usual (Figure 24.1).

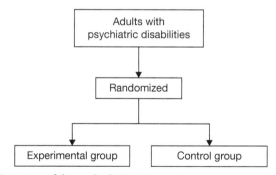

Figure 24.1. Overview of the study design.

Study Intervention: The Bridge Program was a 6-week group intervention, convening twice per week for 2 hours each session (12 sessions total). The

Bridge Program included the following skill-building modules: education/career research, studying, reading, writing, math, computer literacy, library utilization, public speaking, professionalism, socialization, and stress management. Each week participants also met individually with occupational therapy (OT) students for an additional 1 hour. Individualized mentorship addressed volitional strategies, skill application, personalized goal exploration, program application support, study skills, and strategy development to support formal educational participation or employment. OT students facilitated the modules and conducted the mentorship with faculty guidance.

The control group received treatment as usual at their mental health facilities (i.e., medication management, case management, group counseling, and daily activity groups) for 6 weeks.

Follow-Up: Follow-up data collection was reported at both 1 month and 6 months post-treatment.

Endpoints: The study did not designate a primary outcome; effectiveness of the Bridge Program was determined by the following outcomes:
- Application or enrollment in an educational or job training program post-intervention
- Professionalism and social skills required for success in an academic environment (Task Skills Scale, Interpersonal Skills Scale, and School Behavior Scale)
- Participant comfort as an adult learner (Participant Comfort with the Student Role Scale)
- Modular knowledge acquisition (pre- and posttests developed by study authors of the 12 academic modules)

RESULTS

- In the experimental group, 76% of participants completed the Bridge Program (including completion of the 12 modules and mentoring sessions).
- After 6-month follow-up, 63% of participants who completed the Bridge Program either attained paid employment ($n = 1$), enrolled in a college course ($n = 2$), applied to college ($n = 1$), enrolled in an adult education course at a community center ($n = 2$), completed the General Education Development application and prep course ($n = 2$), or enrolled in a technical training certification program ($n = 2$) compared to one

participant (6%) in the control group who enrolled in an educational program.

- Significant differences were captured between the experimental and control group participants' posttest scores on four outcome measures: Participant Comfort with the Student Role Scale, Task Skills Scale, Interpersonal Skills Scale, School Behavior Scale (all $p \leq 0.000$).
- Pre-and posttest scores for each of the 12 modules completed within the Bridge Program demonstrated significant differences, indicating positive learning outcomes.
- Success factors that correlated with program completion and progress in educational or employment goals included adherence to medication routine ($p \leq 0.000$), maintaining stable residence ($p < 0.001$), and consistent program attendance ($p \leq 0.000$).
- Qualitative data gathered from the Participant Overall Satisfaction Scale indicated that Bridge Program participants felt better prepared for further education and job pursuit through skill attainment developed throughout the intervention.
- OT students demonstrated significantly increased comfort levels ($p < 0.01$) when working with individuals with mental illnesses after exposure to this population through programmatic experiences.

Criticisms and Limitations: Due to the small sample size, timing of service provision, and follow-up data spanning 6 months, findings may not be generalized to other adults with psychiatric disabilities or to other supported education/employment programs that measure program completion (i.e., graduation or certification) compared to program enrollment.

Other Relevant Studies and Information:

- A review of 50 intervention studies from 1990 to 2017 targeting adults with mental illness revealed that supported employment and education ($n = 13$) had the strongest supported evidence compared to six other categories of OT interventions: psychoeducation, creative occupations, time use, habit development, group approaches, and animal-assisted therapy (Kirsh et al., 2019).
- Supported education interventions that focus on goal-setting, skill development, cognitive training, and student-directed planning are associated with improvements in educational/vocational attainment,

academic skills, self-esteem, self-determination, and quality of life (Keptner & McCarthy, 2020; Spencer et al., 2018).

- While there are a variety of means for occupational therapists (OTs) to support adults with mental illness in higher education(i.e., disability centers, academic success centers, student health centers, assistive technology centers, transition teams, undergraduate education), supported education programs are the most documented service designs (Keptner & McCarthy, 2020; Spencer et al., 2018).

Summary and Implications: An OT-informed supported education program, created to support adults with psychiatric disabilities, demonstrated significant outcomes in educational and vocational program enrollment, professionalism and social skills, and comfort in the student role. OTs have a unique role in contributing to the attainment, maintenance, and fulfillment of student and worker roles, particularly for people diagnosed with mental illness. As OTs become more involved in supported education and supported employment programs, adults with psychiatric disabilities will have increased opportunities for independence, optimal engagement in society, and acquisition of meaningful habits, routines, and roles.

CLINICAL CASE: STRATEGIES FOR SUCCEEDING IN POSTSECONDARY EDUCATION WITH SCHIZOPHRENIA

Case History

Omari (he/him), a 23-year-old male, comes to the outpatient mental health clinic inquiring about how he can return to community college after a 2-year leave of absence for a previous hospitalization due to schizophrenia. He presents with low self-esteem, low self-efficacy related to his studying skills, and inconsistent medication adherence due to his dislike of the side effects. His sensory profile reveals that he is easily distracted and experiences overstimulation by novel, sensory rich environments. He exhibits proficient reading, writing, and computer skills but experiences difficulty managing anxiety when faced with a multistep task or when needing to speak with faculty. Omari is a motivated and dedicated learner who wants to pursue higher education to advance his passions in computer science.

Suggested Answer

OTs could begin by addressing medication management skills as the Gutman et al. study highlights medication adherence as a significant success factor that correlated with higher education enrollment for clients with psychiatric disabilities. Then, after analyzing barriers to formal education participation, OTs could develop compensatory strategies in collaboration with Omari to address specific client-centered goals, as demonstrated by the individualized mentoring component of the study. The client may benefit from review of modular topics, outlined by the study, emphasizing studying, time management, professional behaviors, and stress management. Suggested intervention includes providing education and skill-building in environmental modifications to optimize concentration, task analyses to break down large assignments, role-playing anxiety-provoking scenarios with professors, and implementing stress-reduction techniques such as meditation, exercise, and leisure.

References

Keptner, K. M., & McCarthy, K. (2020). Mapping occupational therapy practice with postsecondary students: A scoping review. *The Open Journal of Occupational Therapy, 8*(1), 1–17.

Kirsh, B., Martin, L., Hultqvist, J., & Eklund, M. (2019). Occupational therapy interventions in mental health: A literature review in search of evidence. *Occupational Therapy in Mental Health, 35*(2), 109–156.

Spencer, B., Sherman, L., Nielsen, S., & Thormodson, K. (2018). Effectiveness of occupational therapy interventions for students with mental illness transitioning to higher education: A systematic review. *Occupational Therapy in Mental Health, 34*(2), 151–164.

25

Recovering Energy through Nutrition and Exercise for Weight Loss (RENEW)

An Effective Weight Loss Program for People Living with Serious Mental Illness

SOYOUNG ESTHER BAE

Obesity presents challenging health problems for individuals with serious mental illness that require effective interventions. This study of the RENEW program provides evidence that individuals with serious mental illness can benefit from weight loss programs.

BROWN, C., GOETZ, J., & HAMERA, E. (2011). Weight loss intervention for people with serious mental illness: a randomized controlled trial of the RENEW program. *Psychiatric Services, 62*(7), 800–802.

Original Paper: https://doi.org/10.1176/ps.62.7.pss6207_0800

Research Question: Does a 12-month multicomponent intervention tailored for individuals living with serious mental illness support weight loss and lifestyle changes?

Funding: The National Institute of Mental Health and Health Management Resources

Year Study Began: 2007

Year Study Published: 2011

Study Location: Kansas City, KS; Las Vegas, NV

Who Was Studied: There were 136 recipients of community mental health services living with serious mental illness taking psychiatric medication and receiving community mental health services at one of four identified programs enrolled in this study.
- 60% White, 34% African American, 6% other
- 39% male

Who Was Excluded: Not noted

How Many Patients: 136 enrolled, 89 remained at 6 months

Study Overview: There were 136 individuals living with serious mental illness enrolled in this study. Participants were categorized by antipsychotic medications taken, stratified by risk of weight gain, and then randomized to either the control or intervention group (Figure 25.1).

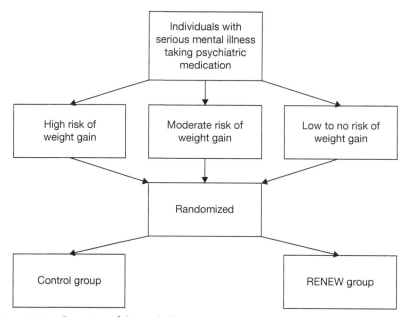

Figure 25.1. Overview of the study design.

Study Intervention: The 12-month intervention consisted of an intensive phase (3 months), a maintenance phase (3 months), and an intermittent support phase (6 months). This study examines the first two phases of the program. In the intensive phase (3 months), participants were provided with weekly 3-hour sessions facilitated by an occupational therapist, dietician, or nurse. Sessions included education about nutrition, opportunities for group-based physical activity, and goal-setting. Social support was an embedded component; a meal was shared during each session. Participants were also given two meal replacements per day for the week. During the maintenance phase (3 months) of the intervention, participants met every month for 3 hours and received weekly support by phone, but no meal replacements were provided. The control group received typical treatment consisting of medication, case management, and optional day programs.

Follow-Up: Weight loss data from the control and intervention groups were gathered at 3 months (immediately following the intensive phase) and 6 months (immediately following the maintenance phase).

Endpoints:

- Primary outcome: differences in weight loss between intervention and control groups at 3 months and 6 months
- Secondary outcome: risk of weight gain by medication category

RESULTS

- Enrolled participants ($n = 136$) were randomized; there were no significant differences in age, race, gender, or weight between the control and intervention groups at baseline.
- At 6 months, 89 evaluable participants remained ($n = 42$ in the RENEW intervention group and $n = 47$ in the control group). There were no significant differences between individuals who completed the study and the 47 individuals who dropped out prior to follow-up.
- At 3 and 6 months, the intervention group had significantly greater weight loss than the control group ($p = 0.005$). At 3 months, the intervention group lost 5.3 pounds, whereas the control group had gained 0.1 pounds; and at 6 months, the intervention group lost 4.4 pounds compared to 0.9 pounds lost in the control group.
- There were no significant differences in weight loss across medication classes associated with different risk of weight gain (Table 25.1).

Table 25.1. OVERVIEW OF THE RENEW STUDY DESIGN

	Intervention Group						Control Group					
	Baseline		3-Month Follow-Up		6-Month Follow-Up		Baseline		3-Month Follow-Up		6-Month Follow-Up	
	M	SD	*M*	SD	*M*	SD	*M*	SD	*M*	SD	*M*	SD
Low risk[a]	224.3	44.1	218.9	43.9	220.9	46.3	255.5	70.1	256.7	68.3	257.8	74.3
Moderate risk[b]	223.3	37.6	219.2	38.1	219.5	41.3	244.0	57.5	242.0	59.7	239.8	56.9
High risk[c]	227.5	50.6	219.8	45.1	220.1	46.4	218.8	47.5	221.2	48.9	219.5	41.3
Total	224.5	41.9	219.2	40.8	220.1	43.3	241.8	60.2	241.9	60.6	240.9	60.5

M = mean; SD = standard deviation.
[a]Low-risk medications: molindone, ziprasidone, fluphenazine, haloperidol, and aripiprazole.
[b]Moderate-risk medications: risperidone, chlorpromazine, quetiapine, and valproate.
[c]High-risk medications: olanzapine, clozapine, and lithium.

Criticisms and Limitations: A large number of participants were lost to follow-up (65% retention rate); thus, results may have been due to attrition bias. The small sample size may have resulted in decreased ability to iden-tify weight loss predictors. The intervention design may not be feasible in all settings, especially the provision of meal replacements during the intensive phase and the staff time required for a 12-month intervention and lengthy (3 hour) weekly/monthly sessions, which may also be taxing for participants, particularly if they are engaging in other productive roles. Lastly, the study lacked information about the program's cultural considerations and about compensatory strategies for cognitive deficits incorporated into the program design.

Other Relevant Studies and Information:

- Following this study, Brown et al. (2014) reported on outcomes after 12 months of the RENEW intervention. Significant variations in response such as variability in weight loss among sites were identified and analyzed. The study suggests that the discrepancy in outcomes may be related to environmental differences (obesogenic environments vs. an established culture of wellness).
- A scoping review found that occupational therapy weight loss interventions based on lifestyle change demonstrate efficacy when delivered in a multimodal format to address increase in activity and

dietary changes. Interventions which combined individual and group sessions were found to have greater success (Conn et al., 2019).

Summary and Implications: The findings of this study reveal that programs that present weight loss strategies within a psychiatric rehabilitation framework can be effective in supporting lifestyle changes that lead to weight loss for individuals living with serious mental illness.

CLINICAL CASE: THE IMPACT OF INTEGRATED HEALTH

Case History

Maya (she/her), a 25-year-old Asian American woman with a diagnosis of schizoaffective disorder, is referred by her psychiatrist to occupational therapy at an outpatient community mental health clinic to address decreased quality of life exacerbated by weight gain. She states that her antipsychotic medication has been causing low energy and hypersomnia, contributing to limited physical activity. Her current body mass index is 32.9, placing her at increased risk for cardiovascular disease and diabetes. What type of intervention should the occupational therapist suggest for this client?

Suggested Answer

Obesity and associated physical health concerns are more commonly found among people with serious mental illness compared to the general population, making them more susceptible to chronic conditions, metabolic syndromes, shorter life expectancy, and lower quality of life. Moreover, obesity rates are found to be even higher in women within this population. As such, effective interventions such as the RENEW program that address weight loss are needed in mental health settings. This study indicates that weight loss programs designed for people with serious mental illness that incorporate both physical activity and dietary changes can be effective in supporting moderate weight loss and maintenance for up to 6 months. Maya may benefit from an intervention that provides weight loss strategies in addition to skill training, goal-setting, and opportunities for social support to address current risk factors. Additionally, her team may want to consider identifying resources for continued support within the clinic or in the community as the RENEW program tapers off.

References

Brown, C., Goetz, J., Hamera, E., & Gajewski, B. (2014). Treatment response to the RENEW weight loss intervention in schizophrenia: Impact of intervention setting. *Schizophrenia Research, 159*(2–3), 421–425.

Conn, A., Bourke, N., James, C., & Haracz, K. (2019). Occupational therapy intervention addressing weight gain and obesity in people with severe mental illness: A scoping review. *Australian Occupational Therapy Journal, 66*(4), 446–457.

26

Occupation-Based Interventions for Addictive Disorders

CARLOS JUAREZ AGUILAR

Occupation-based interventions—that is, interventions that incorporate the performance of an occupation—in the areas of work, leisure and social participation have been used to treat substance related and addictive disorders. . . . Integrating occupation-based interventions in individuals' lives may elicit small but significant improvements in recovery from substance related and addictive disorders.

WASMUTH, S., PRITCHARD, K., & KANESHIRO, K. (2016). Occupation-based intervention for addictive disorders: A systematic review. *Journal of Substance Abuse Treatment, 62,* 1–9.

Original Paper: https://doi.org/10.1016/j.jsat.2015.11.011

Research Question: In persons with addictive disorders, are occupation-based interventions more effective than treatment as usual in improving short-term and long-term recovery outcomes?

Funding: Not applicable

Year Study Began: Not available

Year Study Published: 2016

Study Location: Indianapolis, IN

Who Was Studied: Randomized controlled trials (RCTs) and quasi-controlled trials (QCT) examining occupation-based interventions delivered by a range of addiction rehabilitation disciplines that included five or more participants with substance use disorders.

Who Was Excluded: Studies examining interventions with no activity component.

How Many Studies: 26

Study Overview: Research through database search and other methods yielded 1,099 studies, of which 1,095 were screened after removing duplicates. Of these studies, 170 were assessed for eligibility, with 26 of them meeting criteria for inclusion (see Figure 26.1).

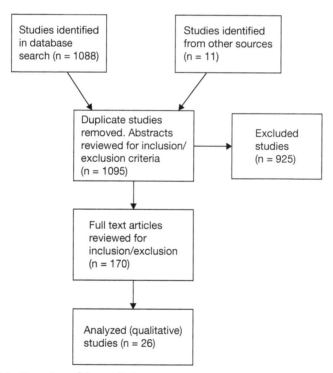

Figure 26.1. Overview of the study design.

Study Intervention: The interventions utilized in each study included in this review were highly variable. Overall, the studies included occupation-based interventions in the areas of work, leisure, or social participation and their impact on people with alcohol, tobacco, cannabis, and/or opiate addictions. Commonly used interventions were yoga, exercise (walking, exercise bike, rower), psychodrama, and music therapy (improvisation, songwriting, music bingo, lyric analysis).

Control group interventions, referred to in this study as "didactic interventions," included group and individual psychotherapy, cognitive-behavioral therapy (CBT), jail diversion, cognitive distraction, and other unspecified treatment as usual.

Follow-Up: Follow-up varied across the 26 studies, ranging from 1 day to 3 months.

Endpoints:

- Substance use outcomes, including self-report of use and craving, urine or saliva analysis of use, diagnostic interviews for substance use disorders, and standardized measures of addictive disorder symptoms, related problems, and readiness to change.
- Symptom severity, measured by standardized symptom measures including the Addiction Severity Index, the Revised Symptom Checklist-90, the Brief Symptom Inventory, and the Circumstances, Motivation, and Readiness Scales for Substance Abuse Treatment.

RESULTS

- Leisure occupations were the most common areas of occupation-based intervention utilized, with 20 studies identified. These interventions yielded a mix of outcomes, with significant between-group differences found in 13 studies, in the domains of drug and alcohol consumption as well as psychiatric and medical status, and no significant differences found in 7 studies (Table 26.1).
- In comparison to psychotherapy, multidimensional family therapy elicited significantly better treatment retention, lower prevalence of cannabis use disorder, and, in heavy users, significantly fewer consumption days than those in the psychotherapy control group.
- Sacks et al. (2012) found a prison therapeutic community to be more effective in reducing drug use, criminal activity, exposure to crime, and reincarceration in female inmates with substance use disorders than CBT.
- Tobacco use disorder was treated solely with exercise, and significant outcomes were largely short term and immediate.

- Opiate use disorder was treated solely with yoga or other similar body–mind interventions such as tai-chi.
- The second most common area used in intervention was that of social participation, with five studies identified. All social participation interventions produced significant between-group differences in treatment retention, drug and alcohol consumption, exposure to crime, criminal activity, and mental health functioning.
- Work occupations were used as an intervention in one study, in which significant between-group differences were found in the areas of drug and alcohol consumption as well as psychiatric and medical status when compensated work therapy was compared to a control group receiving treatment as usual.

Table 26.1. OUTCOMES OF OCCUPATION-BASED INTERVENTIONS
BY TYPE OF STUDY

Outcome	RCT Kashner et al. ($n = 142$)	Shaffer ($n = 61$)	Smelson ($n = 102$)	QCT Rowe et al. ($n = 114$)
Addiction Severity Index				
Family	Not measured	No significant difference	Not measured	Not measured
Employment	Not measured	No significant difference	Not measured	Not measured
Drug consumption	0.08 (−0.32 to 0.48)	No significant difference	Not measured	0 (−0.48 to 0.48)
Alcohol consumption	0.05 (−0.35 to 0.44)	No significant difference	Not measured	0.05 (−0.43 to 0.53)
Psychiatric symptoms	0.16 (−0.24 to 0.56)	No significant difference	Not measured	Not measured
Medical status	0.21 (−0.19 to 0.61)	No significant difference	Not measured	Not measured
	Russell et al. ($n = 42$)	Albornoz et al. ($n = 24$)	Sacks et al. ($n = 468$)	Vedamuthachar et al. ($n = 60$)
Beck Depression Inventory	Not measured	0.10 (−0.70 to 0.90)	0.01 (−0.18 to 0.20)	0.24 (−0.27 to 0.75)

Criticisms and Limitations: The distinction between occupation-based interventions and didactic interventions was not consistent from one study to another, nor did interventions focus on populations that were strictly being treated for addiction. Some interventions involved largely didactic methods with a small occupation-based component. This presents a challenge in translating findings into practice for current treatment programs as it is difficult to discern what was most helpful and what was not.

Other Relevant Studies and Information:

- Similar systematic reviews yielded strong evidence for the benefits of psychoeducation and occupation- and cognitive-based interventions in people with serious mental illness, a population which often overlaps with the addictive disorders population (D'Amico et al., 2018).
- A systematic review of meaningful occupation-based interventions for people living with dementia found that providing meaningful or individualized tailored activities (in other words, occupation-based interventions) for people with dementia living in residential aged care facilities appears to be effective for a range of behavioral and psychological symptoms (Travers et al., 2016).
- A systematic review of occupational therapy's role in the treatment of addiction found low levels of evidence and small sample sizes among 30 studies reviewed. The authors concluded that the research that has been published on this topic is poor (Rojo-Mota et al., 2017).
- An article utilizing 10 semi-structured interviews of people with addiction(s) explored the concept of addiction as occupation. Findings suggest that further research of experiences of addiction as occupation could be useful for informing occupational therapy interventions for substance-related and addictive disorders (Wasmuth et al., 2014).

Summary and Implications:

- Incorporating occupation-based interventions, specifically in the areas of leisure, work, and social participation, may be more effective than treatment as usual alone for treating addictive disorders. The work, leisure, and social participation activities included in this review were low-cost, non-invasive, and accessible. The nature of the occupation-based interventions reviewed by this study suggests that such interventions may be easily integrated into the daily lives of those seeking treatment.

CLINICAL CASE: OCCUPATIONAL PERFORMANCE INTERVENTIONS FOR SUBSTANCE USE DISORDERS

Case History

Sol (they/them) a 34-year-old individual diagnosed with schizophrenia, lives in a supported housing facility for individuals involved in the legal system. They have a history of homelessness, psychiatric hospitalizations, and addiction to methamphetamines. The client has limited contact with their family and often laments not being a part of their two daughters' lives. The client reports that before the onset of symptoms, they were heavily engaged in creating art and had plans to pursue a degree and career in the field.

After weeks of treatment as usual (CBT, psychotherapy, case management, sessions with a substance use counselor) and reporting no significant symptoms of psychosis, Sol leaves the mental health facility and travels to an unknown location to purchase and consume methamphetamines, where they overdose and are hospitalized. Upon return to the supported housing facility, the treatment team meets to discuss potential interventions. How might occupation-based interventions assist this person's recovery?

Suggested Answer

The results of this systematic review indicate that engagement in work, leisure, and social participation occupations may be more effective than treatment as usual alone for individuals with substance use disorders. The occupational therapist could assist Sol in identifying meaningful activities of interest within these occupational performance areas, with the understanding that social participation activities are especially likely to be beneficial.

The client may be encouraged to engage in leisure activities tailored to their particular interests, in this case oil painting. Rather than only presenting information about the benefits of social participation, facilitating social participation activities of interest to the client (playing dominos, joining a basketball team, and attending group Bible studies) is likely to be more beneficial. Finally, engaging Sol in activities that would aid in reconnecting with their family, such as letter-writing, creating art pieces for them, or facilitating phone and video conversations with them, is likely to have a more beneficial effect when incorporated with treatment as usual.

References

Albornoz, Y. (2011). The effects of group improvisational music therapy on depression in adolescents and adults with substance abuse: A randomized controlled trial. *Nordic Journal of Music Therapy*, 20(3), 208–224.

D'Amico, M. L., Jaffe, L. E., & Gardner, J. A. (2018). Evidence for interventions to improve and maintain occupational performance and participation for people with serious mental illness: A systematic review. *American Journal of Occupational Therapy,* 72(5), 7205190020p1–7205190020p11. https://doi.org/10.5014/ajot.2018.033332

Kashner, T. M., Rosenheck, R., Campinell, A. B., Suris, A., Crandall, R., Garfield, N. J., . . . Wicker, A. (2002). Impact of work therapy on health status among homeless, substance-dependent veterans: A randomized controlled trial. *Archives of General Psychiatry,* 59(10), 938–944. http://dx.doi.org/10.1001/archpsyc.59.10.938

Rojo-Mota, G., Pedrero-Pérez, E. J., & Huertas-Hoyas, E. (2017). Centennial topics—Systematic review of occupational therapy in the treatment of addiction: Models, practice, and qualitative and quantitative research. *American Journal of Occupational Therapy,* 71, 7105100030p1–7105100030p11. https://doi.org/10.5014/ajot.2017.022061

Rowe, M., Bellamy, C., Baranoski, M., Wieland, M., O'Connell, M. J., Benedict, P., Davidson, L., Buchanan, J., & Sells, D. (2007). A peer-support, group intervention to reduce substance use and criminality among persons with severe mental illness. *Psychiatric Services (Washington, D.C.),* 58(7), 955–961. https://doi.org/10.1176/ps.2007.58.7.955

Russell, P. O., Epstein, L. H., Johnston, J. J., Block, D. R., & Blair, E. (1988). The effects of physical activity as maintenance for smoking cessation. *Addictive Behaviors,* 13(2), 215–218. https://doi.org/10.1016/0306-4603(88)90016-0

Sacks, J., Mckendrick, K., & Hamilton, Z. (2012). A randomized clinical trial of a therapeutic community treatment for female inmates: Outcomes at 6 and 12 months after prison release. *Journal of Addictive Diseases,* 31, 258–269. https://doi.org/10.1080/10550887.2012.694601

Shaffer, H. J., LaSalvia, T. A., & Stein, J. P. (1997). Comparing Hatha yoga with dynamic group psychotherapy for enhancing methadone maintenance treatment: A randomized clinical trial. *Alternative Therapies in Health and Medicine, 3,* 57–67.

Smelson, D., Kalman, D., Losonczy, M. F., Kline, A., Sambamoorthi, U., Hill, L. S., Castles-Fonseca, K., & Ziedonis, D. (2012). A brief treatment engagement intervention for individuals with co-occurring mental illness and substance use disorders: Results of a randomized clinical trial. *Community Mental Health Journal,* 48(2), 127–132. https://doi.org/10.1007/s10597-010-9346-9

Travers, C., Brooks, D., Hines, S., O'Reilly, M., McMaster, M., He, W., MacAndrew, M., Fielding, E., Karlsson, L., & Beattie, E. (2016). Effectiveness of meaningful occupation interventions for people living with dementia in residential aged care: A systematic review. *JBI Database of Systematic Reviews and Implementation Reports,* 14(12), 163–225. https://doi.org/10.11124/JBISRIR-2016-003230

Vedamurthachar, A., Janakiramaiah, N., Hegde, J. M., Shetty, T. K., Subbakrishna, D. K., Sureshbabu, S. V., & Gangadhar, B. N. (2006). Antidepressant efficacy and hormonal effects of Sudarshana Kriya Yoga (SKY) in alcohol dependent individuals. *Journal of Affective Disorders,* 94(1-3), 249–253. https://doi.org/10.1016/j.jad.2006.04.025

Wasmuth, S., Crabtree, J. L., & Scott, P. J. (2014). Exploring addiction-as-occupation. *British Journal of Occupational Therapy,* 77(12), 605–613.

SECTION 5

Children and Youth

Occupational therapy (OT) with children and youth is multifaceted as it includes a developmental span of 18 years, a variety of practice areas, and distinct disorders with many intervention approaches. This practice area has led the profession in the development of standardized, norm-referenced assessments and the crafting of interventions designed to improve developmental abilities. Given this storied history, we sought to select research studies that reflect the chronological progression of the field, beginning with Ayres. Given the limited number of studies that appear in this volume, we focused our selection on seminal works that have shaped the ways pediatric OT practitioners work today.

Assessment tools targeting specific age groups and a variety of functional problems have played a pivotal role in research and practice within pediatric OT. Three are reviewed in this section: the Sensory Profile (Dunn & Brown) is one of the most often utilized clinical and research tools to identify sensory processing disorders spanning from early childhood to adulthood; the Pediatric Evaluation of Disability Inventory (Haley et al.) assesses functional performance and has been used as an outcome measure in research (Schaaf et al., 2014); and the Test of Playfulness measures an important occupational area in children: play (Harkness & Bundy).

Pediatric OT practice spans from the neonatal period to adolescence, during which time a child builds motor, sensory, cognitive, emotional, social, and adaptive skills; and we sought to choose articles representing this age span. Field et al.'s article on neonatal interventions represents the youngest age group OT practitioners address and has generated a rich area of research and practice (Pineda et al., 2012, 2019). Law et al.'s study, one of the few focusing on older children, addresses environmental barriers to participation for children up to 14 years.

Several articles represent diverse practice areas. Eliasson et al.'s study on constraint-induced movement therapy in young children with hemiplegic cerebral palsy represents a specific approach with consistently positive results that has been utilized with both children and adults with neuromotor disorders. Lawlor and Mattingly's article on family-centered care illustrates the need for adopting a care model that includes shared decision-making between families and service providers. The two articles have contributed to practice differently—the former as a targeted recommendation for a specific population and the latter providing a general viewpoint for practice.

We sought to represent a variety of developmental disorders and intervention approaches by selecting articles that addressed sensory processing disorders and sensory integration treatment practices (Ayres, Miller et al.), cerebral palsy and other neuromotor disorders (Eliasson et al., Harkness & Bundy, Law et al.), and autism (Baranek). These six articles cover some of the most common diagnoses seen in pediatric clinical practice.

In our search, we found that sensory processing and sensory integration were central themes running through OT practice with children and youth. Ayres's article, conducted among children with learning disabilities, is an example of early research on an intervention approach—sensory integration treatment—that continues to be one of the most utilized interventions in pediatric practice (Benson et al., 2019). Ayres's seminal study opened the door to a popular arena of practice, school-based practice; a novel class of disorders, sensory processing disorders; and a new intervention approach, sensory integration treatment. In the tradition of Ayres, Miller et al. is one of the first systematic studies to apply Ayres's intervention to a different population (children with sensory modulation disorders) than was originally studied, which continues to be researched up to the present day (Andelin et al., 2021). Baranek applied a novel retrospective method to the understanding of early signs of autism. Her research was groundbreaking, starting a tradition of research on early signs of autism and their relationship to sensory processing (Flanagan et al., 2012).

Two articles focus on the relationship between the environment and performance: Law et al. identified the barriers to participation in children with developmental disabilities, while Cermak et al. altered the environment in a non-traditional area of practice, the dental clinic, to impact autistic children's participation in teeth cleaning. Both articles emphasize the need for attending to the effect of the environment on participation and, in doing so, broaden the impact of OT.

In identifying studies to include in this volume, we noted that several important topics have limited representation in the literature. For instance, few studies have focused on adolescents, non-White, or non-English-speaking populations. The dearth of studies in these areas points to the need for OT researchers to tackle them in the future. While we faced difficult choices in selecting studies from within the extensive pediatric literature, we hope that this sampling of articles represents the breadth, depth, and richness of this practice area.

References

Andelin, L., Schoen, S., & Reynolds, S. (2021). Effectiveness of occupational therapy using a sensory integration approach: A multiple-baseline design study. *The American Journal of Occupational Therapy, 75*(6), 76–85.

Benson, J. D., Breisinger, E., & Roach, M. (2019). Sensory-based intervention in the schools: A survey of occupational therapy practitioners. *Journal of Occupational Therapy, Schools, & Early Intervention, 12*(1), 115–128.

Flanagan, J. E., Landa, R., Bhat, A., & Bauman, M. (2012). Head lag in infants at risk for autism: A preliminary study. *American Journal of Occupational Therapy, 66*(5), 577–585.

Pineda, R., Raney, M., & Smith, J. (2019). Supporting and enhancing NICU sensory experiences (SENSE): Defining developmentally-appropriate sensory exposures for high-risk infants. *Early Human Development, 133*, 29–35.

Pineda, R. G., Stransky, K. E., Rogers, C., Duncan, M. H., Smith, G. C., Neil, J., & Inder, T. (2012). The single-patient room in the NICU: Maternal and family effects. *Journal of Perinatology, 32*(7), 545–551.

Schaaf, R. C., Benevides, T., Mailloux, Z., Faller, P., Hunt, J., Van Hooydonk, E., . . . & Kelly, D. (2014). An intervention for sensory difficulties in children with autism: A randomized trial. *Journal of Autism and Developmental Disorders, 44*(7), 1493–1506.

27

Hyporesponsiveness to Vestibular Input and Academic Performance

ERNA I. BLANCHE AND SHARON A. CERMAK

Response to Sensory Integration Therapy (SIT)

A larger number of experimental children than control children with hyporeactive nystagmus made greater academic gains. It is concluded that a certain type of vestibular disorder interferes with academic achievement and can be ameliorated through sensory integrative therapy.

AYRES, A. J. (1978). Learning disabilities and the vestibular system. *Journal of Learning Disabilities, 11*(1), 30–41.

Original Paper: https://doi.org/10.1177%2F002221947801100104

Research Question: What neural conditions, specifically response to vestibular input as measured by the Southern California Postrotary Nystagmus Test (SCPNT), predispose a child with learning disabilities to be responsive to sensory integration therapy (SIT), and which measures of sensorimotor and language functions can be used to assess the link to vestibular functions?

Funding: Center for the Study of Sensory Integrative Dysfunction and The Valentine-Kline Foundation

Year Study Began: Not available

Year Study Published: 1978

Study Location: Los Angeles, CA

Who Was Studied: Six- to 10-year-old children diagnosed with learning disabilities. The diagnosis of learning disabilities was based on academic achievement below intellectual ability and inability to benefit from standard education.

Who Was Excluded: Children without learning disorders.

How Many Patients: 92

Study Overview: See Figure 27.1.

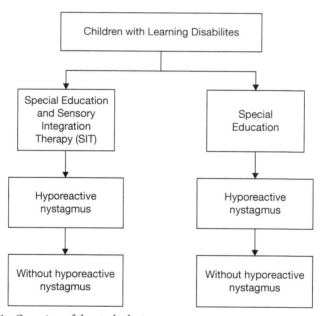

Figure 27.1. Overview of the study design.

Study Intervention: The treatment group received traditional special education in the classroom plus individualized SIT 5 days per week for 30 minutes per day for 6 months, individually or in pairs. Intervention entailed the use of vestibular, tactile, and proprioceptive inputs.

The control group continued with special education in the classroom setting.

Follow-Up: 6 months (immediately following intervention completion)

Endpoints:

- Motor planning and the ability to copy simple figures as measured by the Motor Accuracy Test and the Design Copying Test of Southern California Sensory Integration Tests
- Language abilities and selective attention as measured by the dichotic listening and auditory-language subtests of the Test of Psycholinguistic Abilities
- Auditory processing, as measured by the Flowers-Costello Test of Central Auditory Abilities
- General academic ability, as measured by the Wide Range Achievement Test (WRAT)
- Language ability, as measured by the Slosson Oral Reading Test

Primary and secondary outcomes were not specified.

RESULTS

- Children with learning disabilities who are hyporesponsive to vestibular input as measured with the SCPNT made better gains with SIT and special education than children who were not hyporesponsive to vestibular input. Response to treatment was measured with the WRAT and the dichotic listening test.
- Children who were hyporesponsive to vestibular input also benefited less from special education alone than children who were hyperresponsive to vestibular input or exhibited an average SCPNT.
- Children who are hyporesponsive to vestibular input as measured with the SCPNT performed better in language, academic performance, and sensory-motor tests than children who were hyperresponsive to vestibular input.
- Children with increased scores on the SCPNT exhibited more severe sensory-motor difficulties in motor planning, somatosensory perception, postural control, bilateral motor coordination, visual perception, and auditory-language processes.
- Ayres observed that children who are hyperresponsive to vestibular input appeared to have more generalized difficulties and were less responsive to SIT.

- Decreased response to vestibular input as measured with the SCPNT is a good predictor of academic success following SIT.

Criticisms and Limitations: Participants were not randomized to experimental and control groups, limiting the ability to draw causal inferences from the study's findings. The article includes a minimal description of the intervention, limiting the potential for replicability.

Other Relevant Studies and Information:

- Ayres (1972, 1977) provided the framework for the current study and identified different sensory integration clusters and factors, setting the groundwork for this study.
- de Quiros (1976) described the importance of the vestibular system to language in children with learning disabilities, setting the groundwork for this study.
- Miller et al. (2007) and Schaaf et al. (2014) continued to conduct research on the effectiveness of sensory integration treatment, as first exemplified with this study. However, neither of these contemporary authors examined which specific sensory integration problems respond best to SIT.

Summary and Implications: Children with learning disabilities and shortened duration of postrotary nystagmus (PRN) benefit more from SIT than those with prolonged or average PRN. This is one of the first intervention studies in sensory integration, providing a template to study the effects of SIT and documenting the importance of the vestibular system in predicting response to therapy. Furthermore, it emphasizes the importance of examining not just "Does therapy work?" but rather "For whom does therapy work?"—which remains an important issue for researchers and clinicians today.

CLINICAL CASE: CHILD WHO IS HYPORESPONSIVE TO VESTIBULAR INPUT

Case History

Diego (he/him), a 7-year-old boy, is referred to occupational therapy because he is fidgety, constantly stands up in class, does not pay attention, and reverses letters. Records also show that his academic performance is falling behind. The parents speak Spanish at home. Diego was a late talker who required a speech and language evaluation; however, services were not recommended as the delay was attributed to the child being bilingual. He also had difficulty learning to ride a bike and needed training wheels until he was 6 years old. The teachers and the parents are puzzled about Diego's behavior as his intelligence is above average and he has many friends, but he is not able to do jumping jacks in gym class and does not like participating in sports with balls.

Suggested Answer
The occupational therapist administers a parent questionnaire focusing on sensory processing, a standardized test assessing sensorimotor abilities, the Postrotary Nystagmus Test, and skilled observations focusing on postural control and bilateral motor coordination. The parent report describes Diego as a child who is constantly in motion, while the standardized test of sensorimotor functions together with the skilled observations identify him as someone with decreased postural control, difficulty with bilateral motor coordination, and a shortened duration of PRN. These results indicate that Diego is hyporesponsive to vestibular input, which may contribute to decreased attention, delayed language acquisition, and academic difficulties.

References

Ayres, A. J. (1972). Improving academic scores through sensory integration. *Journal of Learning Disabilities, 5*, 338–343.

Ayres, A. J. (1977). Cluster analyses of measures of sensory integration. *American Journal of Occupational Therapy, 31*(6), 362–366.

de Quiros, J. B. (1976). Diagnosis of vestibular disorders in the learning disabled. *Journal of Learning Disabilities, 9*(1), 39–47.

Miller, L. J., Coll, J. R., & Schoen, S. A. (2007). A randomized controlled pilot study of the effectiveness of occupational therapy for children with sensory modulation disorder. *American Journal of Occupational Therapy, 61*(2), 228–238.

Schaaf, R. C., Benevides, T., Mailloux, Z., Faller, P., Hunt, J., Van Hooydonk, E., Freeman, R., Leiby, B., Sendecki, J., & Kelly, D. (2014). An intervention for sensory difficulties in children with autism: A randomized trial. *Journal of Autism and Developmental Disorders, 44*(7), 1493–1506.

28

Autism during Infancy

STEFANIE BODISON AND ALISON E. LANE

This study confirms that measures of sensory-motor functioning, in addition to indicators of social responsiveness, have potential as early markers of autism during infancy.

BARANEK, G. T. (1999). Autism during infancy: A retrospective video analysis of sensory-motor and social behaviors at 9–12 months of age. *Journal of Autism and Developmental Disorders, 29*(3), 213–224.

Original Paper: https://doi.org/10.1023/A:1023080005650

Research Question: Can subtle symptoms of autism be identified during infancy, and if so, what measures would be relevant and sensitive enough to detect these early behavioral manifestations at 9–12 months of age?

Funding: National Institutes of Health/National Institute of Child Health and Human Development, American Occupational Therapy Association, American Psychological Association

Year Study Began: 1994

Year Study Published: 1999

Study Location: University of North Carolina

Who Was Studied: Children with autism ($n = 11$), children with developmental disabilities ($n = 10$), and typically developing children ($n = 11$) whose families had taken high-quality home videos of them between the ages of 9 and 12 months. There were 19 boys and 13 girls.

Who Was Excluded: Children with significant visual, hearing, or physical impairments (e.g., cerebral palsy) and families with poor-quality videos.

How Many Patients: 32

Study Overview: See Figure 28.1.

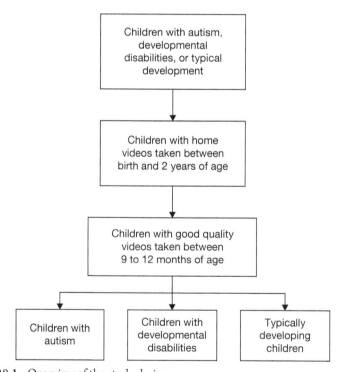

Figure 28.1. Overview of the study design.

Endpoints: The primary outcome was a taxonomy of behaviors observed in the videos to assess across groups and determine which best predicted group status. Nine categories of behaviors were identified and coded: affective expressions, looking, gaze aversion, response to name, social touch responses, anticipatory posture, motor stereotypies, object stereotypes, and sensory modulation.

RESULTS

- Using the retrospective video analysis, nine behaviors (object play, looking at camera, unusual posturing, number of name prompts, orientation to visual stimuli, mouthing of objects, social touch aversions, visual staring/ fixation on objects, and affect rating) were shown to differentiate the groups (children with autism, those with other developmental disorders, and normal children).
- Mouthing, social touch aversions, orientation to visual stimuli, and number of name prompts appeared to discriminate the children with autism from the other groups.
- Posturing, object play rating, looking at camera, visual object stereotypy, and affect rating discriminated the typical children from the children with developmental disabilities and autism.
- Mouthing, orientation to visual stimuli, social touch aversions, posturing, number of name prompts, and affect rating correctly classified children with autism and developmental disabilities at a classification rate of 95%.
- Using these nine behaviors, the classification analysis correctly predicted 93.75% of the cases in the correct diagnostic or typically developing group.

Criticisms and Limitations: One of the most important limitations lies in the inability to standardize the amount of video assessed or the consistency of activities and contexts viewed. The researcher had to use what was available and coded behaviors that were observed. This led to the next limitation: that the video itself provided only a small snippet of time in the child's life and, therefore, was a narrow representation of each child's behaviors.

Other Relevant Studies and Information:

- Subsequent studies have successfully used retrospective video analysis to identify salient sensory-motor behaviors associated with the likelihood of early autism. These behaviors included head lag, use of communicative gestures, and achievement of functional-level object play (Baranek et al., 2005; Flannagan et al., 2012; Watson et al., 2013).
- The consideration of early social and sensory-motor signs together appears to be most accurate in the prediction of autism likelihood in infancy (Baranek et al., 2005; Flannagan et al., 2012; Watson et al., 2013).

Summary and Implications: The results demonstrated that by 9–12 months of age, the pattern of sensory-motor and social behaviors evident in children later diagnosed with autism was contrastingly different from the patterns of behavior demonstrated by neurotypical children and those with developmental disabilities. The results suggest that aspects of sensorimotor functioning, along with measures of social responsiveness, can be used to help identify very young children with autism.

CLINICAL CASE: INFANT EXHIBITING SIGNS OF AUTISM SPECTRUM DISORDER

Case History

Jenny is a 10-month-old child whose older brother, Noah, has a developmental delay and receives school-based occupational therapy services to support his classroom participation. In a recent conversation with Noah's occupational therapist, Jenny's caregiver described several patterns of behaviors that she found worrisome, including Jenny's inability to consistently look at her when her name is called, her excessive mouthing of objects, her desire to watch spinning objects, and her general disregard for social touch. Jenny's caregiver asked if the occupational therapist had any concerns about these behaviors and whether her daughter may be autistic.

Suggested Answer

The occupational therapist explained that some of the behaviors exhibited by Jenny could be signs of autism but that children are not typically diagnosed with autism in infancy. The occupational therapist recommended that Jenny receive a comprehensive evaluation from a developmental pediatrician or neurologist and noted that she may qualify for early intervention services if the evaluation reveals that Jenny has significant delays in achieving developmental milestones. The occupational therapist informed the caregiver that early intervention services would focus on facilitating Jenny's development to support her participation in family life and attainment of developmental milestones.

References

Baranek, G. T., Barnett, C. R., Adams, E. M., Wolcott, N. A., Watson, L. R., & Crais, E. R. (2005). Object play in infants with autism: Methodological issues in retrospective video analysis. *American Journal of Occupational Therapy, 59*(1), 20–30.

Flanagan, J. E., Landa, R., Bhat, A., & Bauman, M. (2012). Head lag in infants at risk for autism: A preliminary study. *American Journal of Occupational Therapy, 66*(5), 577–585.

Watson, L. R., Crais, E. R., Baranek, G. T., Dykstra, J. R., & Wilson, K. P. (2013). Communicative gesture use in infants with and without autism: A retrospective home video study. *American Journal of Speech–Language Pathology, 22*(1), 25–39.

29

Adapting the Environment for Improved Oral Care among Children on the Autism Spectrum

TEAL W. BENEVIDES AND BETH PFEIFFER

SADE Intervention Study

The development of a modified dental environment may therefore be a promising approach to enable greater numbers of pediatric dentists as well as general dentists trained in advanced behavioral guidance techniques to reduce common dental behavior management problems that occur when treating children with ASD.

CERMAK, S. A., STEIN DUKER, L. I., WILLIAMS, M. E., DAWSON, M. E., LANE, C. J., & POLIDO, J. C. (2015). *Sensory adapted dental environments to enhance oral care for children with autism spectrum disorders: A randomized controlled pilot study. Journal of Autism and Developmental Disorders, 45(9), 2876–2888.*

Original Paper: https://doi.org/10.1007/s10803-015-2450-5

Research Question: What are the feasibility and preliminary efficacy of a sensory adapted dental environment (SADE) compared to a regular dental environment (RDE) in decreasing arousal, uncooperative behavior, pain, and sensory discomfort among children with and without autism spectrum disorder (ASD)?

Funding: Seed grant from the University of Southern California Ostrow School of Dentistry; National Institute of Dental and Craniofacial Research; and the Eunice Kennedy Shriver Institute of Child Health and Human Development, National Institutes of Health

Year Study Began: 2012

Year Study Published: 2015

Study Location: Los Angeles, CA

Who Was Studied: Children between the ages of 6 and 12 years with and without ASD participated. Children must have had at least one prior oral dental cleaning and had to speak either English or Spanish.

Who Was Excluded: Children in either group who had motor, genetic, endocrine, or metabolic co-occurring conditions; children in the "typically developing" (TD) group who had siblings with a diagnosis of an ASD.

How Many Patients: 44

Study Overview: This study used a pilot randomized, crossover, two-group, pretest/posttest design (Figure 29.1).

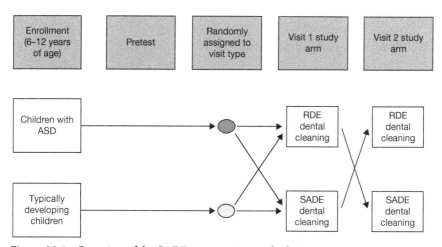

Figure 29.1. Overview of the SADE intervention study design.

Image adapted from Figure 1 of Cermak et al.

Study Intervention: A randomized crossover design was used in which each study group (ASD, TD) received both interventions. The two conditions included a SADE and an RDE. There were no adaptations or changes made in the RDE. The experimental SADE focused on changes to the sensory and physical environment including the following:

- *Visual adaptations* (i.e., clinician using dental head lamp, room-darkening curtains, reduced overhead lighting, and slow-moving visual images projected onto the ceiling)
- *Auditory adaptations* (i.e., music with slow rhythms projected through a speaker)
- *Tactile modifications* (i.e., a weighted dental X-ray shield designed to look like a butterfly to provide deep pressure—all children could request that the wrap be removed if desired so that it was not perceived as a restraint).

Follow-Up: Measures were collected during intervention and immediately following intervention conditions.

Endpoints:

Primary: Child's physiological stress and anxiety (as measured by skin conductance level and non-specific skin conductance responses)

Secondary:

- Child behavioral distress, as measured by
  - o An independent observer's rating on the Children's Dental Behavior Rating Scale
  - o Dentist's rating on the Anxiety and Cooperation Scale and the Frankl Scale
- Child pain intensity (Faces Pain Scale-Revised)
- Child's sensory discomfort (Dental Sensory Sensitivity Scale)
- Cost-savings: length of dental cleaning, number of people needed to restrain, and whether pharmacological intervention (anesthesia) was needed to complete dental cleaning

RESULTS

- The SADE intervention was feasible to implement reliably and acceptable to the children who were enrolled. There were no adverse events reported as a result of the SADE.
- All children (ASD and TD) had statistically lower physiological stress responses with the SADE compared to the RDE, with moderate to large effect sizes.
- Secondary behavioral outcomes did not show statistically significant differences by intervention condition.
- Behavioral effects of the SADE intervention were in the hypothesized direction, meaning that the children with ASD reported less anxiety and less pain and were reported to be calmer by dental practitioners (Table 29.1).
- The SADE did not decrease the amount of time for cleaning, but the number of "hands" needed to restrain the child during a cleaning was less in the SADE than the RDE.

Table 29.1. KEY OUTCOMES

Outcome	Main Effect of Group (TD vs. ASD)	Main Effect of Intervention (RDE vs. SADE)	Interaction Between Group and Environment
Lower electrodermal activity (SCL)	SS, favoring TD	SS, favoring SADE $ES_{ASD} = 0.65$ $ES_{TD} = 0.42$	n.s.
Lower electrodermal activity (NS-SCR)	SS, favoring TD	SS, favoring SADE $ES_{ASD} = 0.27$ $ES_{TD} = 0.30$	n.s.
Lower behavioral distress (three measures)	SS, favoring TD	n.s. for all measures Range $ES_{ASD} = 0.13–0.23$ Range $ES_{TD} = 0.04–0.29$	n.s.
Lower child-rated pain intensity	n.s.	SS, favoring SADE $ES_{ASD} = 0.62$ $ES_{TD} = 0.49$	Not reported
Duration of cleaning	Not reported	SS, favoring RDE $ES_{ASD} = 0.80$ $ES_{TD} = 0.78$	Not reported

SCL = skin conductance level; NS-SCR = non-specific skin conductance response; SS = statistically significant at $p < 0.05$; n.s. = not significant; ES = Cohen's d effect size, calculated within groups only.

Criticisms and Limitations:

- Although the study was designed as a feasibility study and to gather preliminary data on the efficacy of the SADE, effect sizes seemed overstated. According to historical guidelines, the effect size for the TD group is more appropriately categorized as small and that for the ASD group as small to moderate versus moderate to large as described in the article.
- Several of the behavioral outcome measures were created specifically for this study and were not previously validated (e.g., Children's Dental Behavior Rating Scale, Sensory Discomfort Rating Scale). The validity of these measures was not established or examined in this study.
- This study was described as a feasibility study, but limited measures of feasibility were discussed: participant retention, intervention fidelity, and cost. Practitioner-reported feasibility of implementing the SADE was provided in the discussion, but there were not clear measures reported to collect and report this information in the methods or results.

Other Relevant Studies and Information:

- A study examining the environmental impacts on primary care for adults with ASD identified both sensory factors and communication as barriers to primary care encounters. Participants endorsed both patient- and physician-initiated strategies including sensory environmental adaptations, environmental preparation, and scheduling modifications (Stein Duker et al., 2019).
- Emerging literature describes multisensory environments that could be used to address occupational performance difficulties among individuals with intellectual and developmental disabilities (Breslin et al., 2020).
- Among typically developing children, decreasing waiting room time prior to a dental appointment was associated with less dental anxiety, although being in a sensorily adapted waiting room environment did not alter dental anxiety (Fux-Noy et al., 2019).

Summary and Implications: This study demonstrated that SADEs are feasible and have the potential to decrease physiological and behavioral distress for children with ASD and, to a lesser extent, children without ASD during routine dental care. The intervention was low-cost and required little to no training of dental providers, relying instead on environmental adaptations. Future research with larger samples is needed to determine which intervention components are most effective.

CLINICAL CASE: ORAL CARE FOR A CHILD WITH AUTISM AND SENSORY HYPERSENSITIVITY

Case History

Sam (he/him) is a 10-year-old boy with a history of poor oral health. He was referred for dental care at the local university clinic for a routine checkup. His last visit to a dentist was at 7 years of age, when his family reported he had a major "meltdown" and would not let the dentist examine his teeth. At that time, he was rescheduled to complete his routine dental checkup and any dental care required under general anesthesia at a 1-day surgical center, where his teeth were cleaned and he had three cavities filled. Sam has severe tactile and oral hypersensitivities and extreme dental anxiety.

What are important considerations for the dental staff and Sam's family to prepare for the dental visit?

Suggested Answer

Cermak and colleagues highlight a number of potential care considerations for children with and those without ASD who have dental distress and anxiety. There is preliminary evidence that the use of environmental modifications to reduce sensory discomfort and to increase relaxation can lessen potential anxiety and distress. Suggested adaptations include calming music, decreased lighting, and deep-pressure tactile input through a dental X-ray vest. Sam may benefit from these types of environmental modifications during the routine dental checkup, as well as preparatory activities prior to his visit. For example, social stories were used both in the current study and in a number of other healthcare-related studies to prepare patients for routine care procedures.

References

Breslin, L., Guerra, N., Ganz, L., & Ervin, D. (2020). Clinical utility of multisensory environments for people with intellectual and developmental disabilities: A scoping review. *American Journal of Occupational Therapy, 74*(1), 7401205060p1–7401205060p12. https://doi.org/10.5014/ajot.2020.037267

Fux-Noy, A., Zohar, M., Herzog, K., Shmueli, A., Halperson, E., Moskovitz, M., & Ram, D. (2019). The effect of the waiting room's environment on level of anxiety experienced by children prior to dental treatment: A case control study. *BMC Oral Health, 19*(1), 294. https://doi.org/10.1186/s12903-019-0995-y

Stein Duker, L. I., Kim, H. K. S., Pomponio, A., Mosqueda, L., & Pfeiffer, B. (2019). Examining primary care health encounters for adults with autism spectrum disorder. *American Journal of Occupational Therapy, 73*(5), 7305185030p1–7305185030p11.

30

Evaluation of Sensory Processing Using the Sensory Profile Questionnaire

RENEE WATLING AND CRISTIN HOLLAND

Sensory Profile factor analysis

[The finding that factor loadings sort out by the child's responsivity to sensory experiences suggests] that it is important to consider not only which sensory systems are affected, but also how persons tend to respond to stimuli. Therapists can use the factors identified in this study to examine patterns of performance in the children they serve.

DUNN, W., & BROWN, C. (1997). *Factor analysis on the Sensory Profile from a national sample of children without disabilities. American Journal of Occupational Therapy, 51(7), 490–499.*

Original Paper: https://doi.org/10.5014/ajot.51.7.490

Research Question: Examine and identify relationships among the 125 items of the Sensory Profile, a tool designed to assess children's responses to commonly occurring sensory events.

Funding: Maternal and Child Health Bureau, University of Kansas, American Occupational Therapy Foundation

Year Study Began: Not available

Year Study Published: 1997

Study Location: National survey based in Kansas

Who Was Studied: Children without disabilities ages 3–10 who were identified by 166 therapists from across the United States and whose parents completed the Sensory Profile.

Who Was Excluded: Children currently taking regular prescription medication (e.g., for hyperactivity or seizures) or receiving special education services.

How Many Patients: 1037

Study Overview: See Figure 30.1.

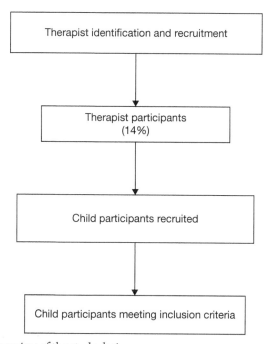

Figure 30.1. Overview of the study design.

Study Intervention: Parents responded to 125 items on the Sensory Profile. The items were designed to investigate behaviors believed to represent a child's sensory processing. Items were arranged in eight categories: auditory, visual, taste/ smell, movement, body position, touch, activity level, and emotional/social. Parents used a 5-point Likert-type scale ranging from *always, when presented with the opportunity, or 100% of the time* to *never, when presented with the opportunity, or 0% of the time*, to report how frequently their child demonstrated the behaviors. The resulting data were used to conduct a principal components factor analysis to determine if the items on the Sensory Profile clustered into meaningful, independent groups. A Varimax orthogonal rotation was used to facilitate interpretation of the analysis.

Follow-Up: Cross-sectional—no follow-up reported.

Endpoints: The primary outcome was an interpretable factor structure for the Sensory Profile that clustered items into meaningful, independent groupings reflecting sensory processing patterns in children.

RESULTS

- The initial factor analysis resulted in 17 factors that accounted for 59.6% of the variance. Eight of the factors were item-specific, having only one or two items with loadings >0.40.
- Items with communalities of <0.40 were eliminated from the analysis; a total of 44 items were eliminated, yielding an 81-item questionnaire.
- After examination, a nine-factor solution that accounted for 47.8% of the variance (see Table 30.1) was deemed to be most interpretable. Items that had loadings ≥0.40 were included in a factor.
- Seventy-five percent of the items had factor loadings >0.50.
- Factors that emerged in this study of children without disabilities are similar to patterns of sensory modulation observable among children with disabilities, suggesting consistency in behaviors indicative of sensory modulation despite disability status.

Note: The Sensory Profile was revised in 2014 using normative data from 2012–2013. The Sensory Profile-2 (Dunn, 2014) includes versions applicable for ages birth through 14 years and can be completed by caregivers or schoolteachers. The Adolescent/Adult Sensory Profile (Brown & Dunn, 2002) can be used for individuals 11 years and older and is completed via self-report.

TABLE 30.1. FACTOR ANALYSIS

Factor Name	Percentage of Variance
Factor 1: Sensory Seeking	22.2
Factor 2: Emotionally Reactive	6.1
Factor 3: Low Endurance/Tone	4.0
Factor 4: Oral Sensory Sensitivity	3.3
Factor 5: Inattention/Distractibility	2.7
Factor 6: Poor Registration	2.6
Factor 7: Sensory Sensitivity	2.5
Factor 8: Sedentary	2.3
Factor 9: Fine Motor/Perceptual	2.1

Criticisms and Limitations: While the researchers describe their methods as a principal components factor analysis, principal component analysis (PCA) and factor analysis are two different statistical approaches. PCA should not be used to understand latent factors, such as sensory processing patterns, which cannot be measured directly (Widaman, 1993; Preacher & MacCallum, 2003).

Other Relevant Studies and Information:

- The Sensory Profile can discriminate between children with and without disabilities and between children with autism spectrum disorder (ASD) and children with attention deficit hyperactivity disorder (Ermer & Dunn, 1998).
- Additional caregiver-report questionnaires (i.e., the Sensory Processing Measure [Parham et al., 2007]) have been developed to assess sensory processing in children with and without ASD and show convergent validity with the Sensory Profile but may produce different results in who is classified with sensory processing challenges (Brown et al., 2010).
- Scores on the Sensory Profile can be interpreted according to five sensory subtypes that occurred in children with typical development and those with developmental delay diagnoses, suggesting that sensory processing patterns may be more reflective of the ability to respond to environmental demands than indicative of a diagnostic condition (Little et al., 2016).
- Practice guidelines for occupational therapy practitioners working with children and adolescents with sensory processing challenges have been published by the American Occupational Therapy Association (Watling

et al., 2018). These guidelines address approaches to evaluation and include case examples using the Sensory Profile and the Sensory Processing Measure.

Summary and Implications: The Sensory Profile items loaded onto eight factors associated with responsivity to intensity or duration of sensory experiences and one factor associated with fine motor/perceptual function. This differs from the traditional way of gathering information according to the sensory system. The factors found for children without disabilities align with sensory patterns often observed in children with disabilities. This finding suggests that sensory modulation and its effects on daily life ought to be considered in the evaluation and intervention for sensory processing. The Sensory Profile can be used to examine patterns of sensory processing in children with and without identified disabilities.

CLINICAL CASE: EVALUATING A CHILD DEMONSTRATING SENSORY PROCESSING CHALLENGES

Case History

Tan (he/him) is the youngest boy in a family with four other children. During Tan's 4-year well child check, the pediatrician noted that he displayed hyperactivity, poor attention, and clumsiness. Tan's mother reported that he was a picky eater, resisted getting dressed, and rarely played with small toys and games. His mother expressed frustration about his difficulty sitting still and refusal to eat the traditional foods she prepared for family meals. She also felt that Tan needed more supervision than her other children had when they were the same age and that he tended to have emotional outbursts over simple things that did not bother others. The pediatrician referred Tan for an occupational therapy evaluation.

Suggested Answer

The occupational therapist completed a comprehensive evaluation of Tan, including administration of standardized assessments of gross and fine motor skills and activities of daily living, clinical observations of play and eating patterns, and an interview of Tan's mother regarding daily life habits and patterns. Her report of picky eating, limited play, difficulty falling asleep, and general hyperactivity raised red flags about sensory processing. The therapist then had Tan's mother complete the Sensory Profile-2. The information from the Sensory Profile-2 helped the occupational therapist identify challenges in the areas of tactile and vestibular sensory processing, with Tan demonstrating sensitivity and avoidance behaviors in both of these areas. She shared the results with Tan's mother and explained the role of sensory processing in Tan's participation and performance challenges in mealtimes, dressing, and play. Together they collaborated on planning interventions that matched the family's values and aimed to increase his participation and performance. Interventions included having Tan and his mother participate in a clinic-based feeding group to decrease oral tactile sensitivity and increase exposure to food textures frequently incorporated into family meals. Additionally, Tan received individual clinic-based occupational therapy utilizing an Ayres' sensory integration approach to support his ability to modulate responses to tactile and vestibular sensory stimuli, enabling him to participate for a longer duration in mealtime, dressing, and play activities.

References

Brown, C., & Dunn, W. (2002). *Adolescent/adult Sensory Profile manual*. Psychological Corporation.

Brown, T., Morrison, I. C., & Stagnitti, K. (2010). The convergent validity of two sensory processing scales used with school-age children: Comparing the Sensory Profile and the Sensory Processing Measure. *New Zealand Journal of Occupational Therapy*, 57(2), 56–65.

Dunn, W. (2014). *Sensory Profile 2*. Psychological Corporation.

Ermer, J., & Dunn, W. (1998). The Sensory Profile: A discriminant analysis of children with and without disabilities. *American Journal of Occupational Therapy*, 52(4), 283–290. https://doi.org/10.5014/ajot.52.4.283

Little, L. M., Dean, E., Tomchek, S. D., & Dunn, W. (2016). Classifying sensory profiles of children in the general population. *Child: Care, Health, and Development*, 43(1), 81–88.

Parham, L. D., Ecker, C., Miller Kuhaneck, H., Henry, D. A., & Glennon, T. J. (2007). *Sensory processing measure: Home form and main classroom and school environments forms*. Western Psychological Services.

Preacher, K. J., & MacCallum, R. C. (2003). Repairing Tom Swift's electric factor analysis machine. *Understanding Statistics*, 2(1), 13–43.

Watling, R., Miller Kuhaneck, H., Parham, L. D., & Schaaf, R. C. (2018). *Occupational therapy practice guidelines for children and youth with challenges in sensory integration and sensory processing*. AOTA Press.

Widaman, K. F. (1993). Common factor analysis versus principal component analysis: Differential bias in representing model parameters? *Multivariate Behavioral Research*, 28(3), 263–311.

31

An Adapted Model of Constraint-Induced Movement Therapy for Young Children with Hemiplegic Cerebral Palsy

MEGAN C. CHANG AND ARAMEH ANVARIZADEH

The children who received [constraint-induced] therapy improved their ability to use their hemiplegic hand significantly more than the children in the control group after 2 months, i.e. after treatment.

ELIASSON, A. C., KRUMLINDE-SUNDHOLM, L., SHAW, K., & WANG, C. (2005). Effects of constraint-induced movement therapy in young children with hemiplegic cerebral palsy: An adapted model. *Developmental Medicine & Child Neurology*, 47(4), 266–275.

Original Paper: https://doi.org/10.1017/S0012162205000502

Research Question: What are the effects of modified constraint-induced movement therapy (mCIMT) compared to conventional pediatric treatment on bimanual hand use in children with hemiplegic cerebral palsy?

Funding: Department of Habilitation Services for Children and Youth, Research Unit, Stockholm and Stockholm County Council, FOU Committee

Year Study Began: Not available

Year Study Published: 2005

Study Location: Stockholm, Sweden

Who Was Studied: Children aged between 18 months and 4 years of age diagnosed with hemiplegic cerebral palsy with any degree of impaired hand function and able to understand simple instructions participated in the study.

Who Was Excluded: Parents who were not able to make the commitment or children who refused to wear the constraining glove were excluded.

How Many Patients: 45

Study Overview: The intervention group participants were recruited from 13 pediatric service centers in the region of the Stockholm County Council, while the control group participants were mainly recruited from other regions in Sweden (Figure 31.1).

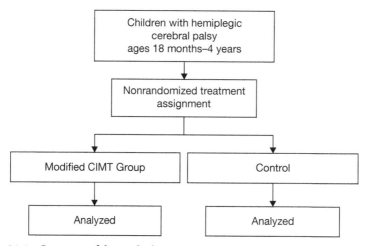

Figure 31.1. Overview of the study design.

Study Intervention: Children in the intervention group received mCIMT from Taub's original CIMT model (Taub et al. 1993, 1999; Taub & Uswatte 2003). These children were expected to wear a restraining glove on the unaffected arm for a total of 2 hours daily for 2 months either at home or at preschool, for a total of 120 hours. Parents and teachers were required to implement the treatment on a daily basis with supervision from a therapist once a week and to enter the treatment time in a logbook.

The children in the control group, matched for age with the intervention group, received conventional pediatric therapy services, which included physical therapy twice per month and occupational therapy once a month.

Follow-Up: Two months (immediately after the intervention) and 6 months after initial assessment.

Endpoints:

- Primary outcome: Hand function when involved in bimanual activity during play measured by Assisting Hand Assessment (AHA; Krumlinde-Sunholm & Eliasson, 2003). The therapists who scored the evaluation results were blinded from the study groups and data collection process.
- Brain imaging information about type of lesion was used to measure whether the type of lesion may influence the ability to obtain benefit from the mCIMT/CI therapy.

RESULTS

- Of the 45 children enrolled in the study, 21 out of 25 in the mCIMT group, and 20 out of 20 in the control group completed the program.
- Children in the mCIMT group significantly improved their affected hand use using the AHA measure compared to children in the control group at the 6-month evaluation ($p = 0.005$).
- The mCIMT group improved the most versus the control group with respect to "reaches," "moves upper arm," and "stabilizes by weight" measured by AHA at 2 months. The control group showed different patterns of change and made less progress overall.
- Regarding factors predictive of the results of treatment:
  - The duration of practice was not correlated to hand function improvement. On average, the child wore the constraining glove for 59 hours of the expected 120 hours of treatment (range 16–120 hours).
  - Baseline hand function was significantly associated with improvement ($r = -0.55$, $p = 0.009$). That is, in both the mCIMT group and the control group, children with more impaired hand function at baseline

improved significantly more than those who started with better hand function.
• Older age was predictive of greater improvement in hand function but only among children in the mCIMT group, with no relationship between age and improvement observed in the control group.

Criticisms and Limitations: Results may not be generalizable to children with other forms of cerebral palsy or to older children. The study did not include a longitudinal follow-up beyond 6 months, so it is not possible to ascertain whether benefits were sustained over time or how the effects transferred to the school setting. The treatment hours and intensity for the mCIMT group varied considerably from 16 to 120 hours due to compliance rate and feasibility for parents and teachers, because of factors such as sickness and lack of staff.

Other Relevant Studies and Information:

• A similar mCIMT study on children aged 18 months to 12 years with unilateral spastic cerebral palsy showed that the mCIMT group significantly improved in hand use during activities after 6 weeks of mCIMT, followed by 2 weeks of bimanual task-specific training, compared to children in a usual rehabilitation care group (Aarts et al., 2010).
• A multicenter, cluster-randomized controlled trial examined the effects of mCIMT compared to bimanual intensive rehabilitation treatment and a traditional rehabilitation program on children with hemiplegic cerebral palsy aged 2–8 years. Findings showed that both the mCIMT and the intensive rehabilitation treatment groups improved significantly relative to the traditional rehabilitation group in paretic hand function (Facchin et al., 2011).
• CIMT treatment has also been shown to significantly improve hand function and attainment of self-determined goals among children 3.5–10 years of age with hemiplegic cerebral palsy (Gordon et al., 2011).

Summary and Implications: Among children with hemiplegic cerebral palsy and impaired hand function, mCIMT improves spontaneous hand function for a variety of activities and is feasible to implement both at home and in school settings. The magnitude of improvement was greatest among older children receiving mCIMT.

CLINICAL CASE: INCORPORATING BOTH UPPER EXTREMITIES DURING FUNCTIONAL TASKS WHEN WORKING WITH YOUNG CHILDREN WITH HEMIPLEGIA

Case History

Angela, a 40-month-old Hispanic girl with right hemiplegic cerebral palsy has been receiving occupational therapy since she was 18 months old. Even though she has now acquired the necessary motor skills to incorporate her right arm in functional tasks, she does not automatically do so. Her occupational therapist reviews the literature searching for ways to enhance the treatment being provided and based on the findings in the Eliasson et al. study, the therapist refers Angela to a mCIMT program at an outpatient clinic.

Suggested Answer

Following assessment, it is determined that Angela is a good candidate, and she is enrolled in a short-term mCIMT program. The therapist at the mCIMT program reviews the intervention program with Angela's mother, describing that the program requires caregivers to commit to a 2-month treatment period during which time the child wears a restraint glove for 2 hours per day. Angela's mother agrees that she can add the 2-hours into her schedule on a daily basis with support from her extended family. While Angela wears the restraint glove, her mother and other caregivers present enjoyable playful activities at the right level of difficulty for Angela to interact with them with her right arm. In addition, the therapist regularly visits Angela to support caregiver training. Angela's mother also keeps a diary documenting the time the glove is worn. All other services remained the same.

After two months participating in the mCIMT program, Angela is reevaluated and found to be consistently incorporating her right arm in bimanual tasks. The parents are thrilled as the program allowed them to carry out the intervention in the home environment and they appreciate Angela's increased use of the affected upper extremity.

References

Aarts, P. B., Jongerius, P. H., Geerdink, Y. A., van Limbeek, J., & Geurts, A. C. (2010). Effectiveness of modified constraint-induced movement therapy in children with unilateral spastic cerebral palsy: A randomized controlled trial. *Neurorehabilitation and Neural Repair, 24*(6), 509–518.

Facchin, P., Rosa-Rizzotto, M., Visonà Dalla Pozza, L., Turconi, A. C., Pagliano, E., Signorini, S., Tornetta, L., Trabacca, A., Fedrizzi, E., & GIPCI Study Group. (2011). Multisite trial comparing the efficacy of constraint-induced movement therapy with that of bimanual intensive training in children with hemiplegic cerebral palsy: Postintervention results. *American Journal of Physical Medicine and Rehabilitation, 90,* 539–553.

Gordon, A. M., Hung, Y.-C., Brandao, M., Ferre, C. L., Kuo, H.-C., Friel, K., Petra, E., Chinnan, A., & Charles, J. R. (2011). Bimanual training and constraint-induced movement therapy in children with hemiplegic cerebral palsy: A randomized trial. *Nuerorehabilitation and Neural Repair, 25*(8), 692–702.

Krumlinde-Sundholm, L., & Eliasson, A. C. (2003). Development of the Assisting Hand Assessment: A Rasch-built measure intended for children with unilateral upper limb impairments. *Scandinavian Journal of Occupational Therapy, 10,* 16–26.

Taub, E., Miller, N. E., Novack, T. A., Cook, E. W., Fleming, W. C., Nepomuceno, C. S., Connell, J. S., & Crago, J. E. (1993). Technique to improve chronic motor deficit after stroke. *Archives of Physical Medicine and Rehabilitation, 74,* 347–354.

Taub, E., & Uswatte, G. (2003). Constraint-induced movement therapy: Bridging from the primate laboratory to the stroke rehabilitation laboratory. *Journal Rehabilitation Medicine, 41*(Suppl), 34–40.

Taub, E., Uswatte, G., Pidikiti, R. (1999). Constraint-induced movement therapy: A new family of techniques with broad application to physical rehabilitation—A clinical review. *Journal of Rehabilitation Research and Development, 36,* 237–251.

32

Moderate- versus Light-Pressure Massage Therapy Leads to Greater Weight Gain in Preterm Infants

LEAH I. STEIN DUKER AND MARSHAE D. FRANKLIN

The moderate pressure massage therapy group gained more weight than the light pressure massage group . . . [and] was more relaxed and less aroused than the light pressure massage therapy group. This was evident in their showing less stressed and more relaxed behavior states . . . and lower heart rate.

> FIELD, T., DIEGO, M. A., HERNANDEZ-REIF, M., DEEDS, O., & FIGUEREIDO, B. (2006). Moderate versus light pressure massage therapy leads to greater weight gain in preterm infants. *Infant Behavior and Development*, 29(4), 574–578.

Original Paper: https://pubmed.ncbi.nlm.nih.gov/17138310/

Research Question: In preterm infants of 28–32 weeks gestational age in the neonatal intensive care unit (NICU), what is the effect of moderate-pressure massage therapy on behavioral states, heart rate, vagal activity, and weight gain compared with light-pressure massage therapy during a 5-day massage therapy intervention?

Funding: National Institutes of Health (National Institute of Mental Health and National Center for Complementary and Alternative Medicine/National Center for Complementary and Integrative Health), March of Dimes, and Johnson & Johnson Pediatric Institute

Year Study Began: Not reported

Year Study Published: 2006

Study Location: Not reported

Who Was Studied: Medically stable preterm infants 28–32 weeks of gestational age with birth weight 550–1800 g, current weight 1000–1900 g, NICU stay 15–60 days, and not receiving antibiotics or phototherapy.

Who Was Excluded: Preterm infants who had genetic anomalies, congenital heart malformations, or central nervous system dysfunction; were HIV-positive; required surgery; or had a history of maternal alcohol/illicit drug use, syphilis, or hepatitis B.

How Many Patients: 68

Study Overview: See Figure 32.1.

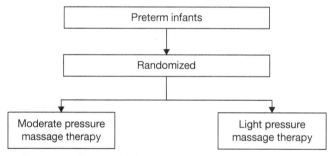

Figure 32.1. Overview of the study design.

Study Intervention: All infants received three 15-minute massages per day for 5 days by trained massage therapists, administered approximately 1 hour after feeding. As explicated in Field et al., massages included 5 minutes each of tactile stimulation, kinesthetic stimulation, and tactile stimulation again. For *tactile stimulation* phases, the infant is prone, and massage strokes are administered in a standardized speed spanning five different body regions. Either moderate-pressure (e.g., slight indentation in skin) or light-pressure stroking is applied based on condition assignment (moderate- vs. light-pressure massage therapy, respectively). In the *kinesthetic stimulation* phase, the infant is supine, and the intervener flexes and extends each arm, each leg, and then both legs together (bicycle motion). The kinesthetic stimulation phase was not changed based on pressure condition.

Follow-Up:

- *Weight*: Measured 2 days prior to intervention and throughout 5-day study.
- *Sleep–wake behaviors, behavior states, and heart rate/vagal tone*: Measured during 15-minute baseline period immediately prior to and throughout 15-minute intervention.

Endpoints:

- *Weight gain*: Measured 2 days prior to intervention and throughout the 5-day study.
- *Sleep–wake behaviors and behavior states (e.g., deep sleep, fussing, crying, movement, hiccupping)*: Reported as percent time during 15 minutes immediately prior to intervention and throughout 15-minute massage therapy intervention.
- *Heart rate*: Reported as beats per minute during 15 minutes immediately prior to intervention and throughout 15-minute massage therapy intervention.

RESULTS

- Significant within-group changes were observed from baseline to during intervention for the following measures (see Table 32.1):
  - o Moderate-pressure group:
    - Improvement in weight gain (5.6 g increase; $p < 0.05$).
    - Improvement in heart rate (6.5 bpm decrease; $p < 0.05$).
  - o Light-pressure group:
    - Decrease in deep sleep (26.6% time decrease; $p < 0.05$).
    - Increase in fussing (16.0% time increase; $p < 0.05$).
    - Increase in crying (9.8% time increase; $p < 0.05$).
    - Increase in movement (8.1% time increase; $p < 0.05$).
    - Increase in stress behavior (hiccupping; 4.8% time increase; $p < 0.01$).

Table 32.1. CHANGES IN NEONATAL MEASURES FROM BEGINNING OF STUDY
TO END OF 5-DAY INTERVENTION PERIOD, BY MODERATE- AND LIGHT-PRESSURE
MASSAGE THERAPY GROUPS

| | Groups | | *p* |
	Moderate	Light	
Change from beginning of study to end of 5-day intervention			
Weight gain (g)	5.6	−0.4	<0.02
Change from baseline to intervention	( )		
Deep sleep (% time)	−3.0	−26.6	<0.05
Active sleep (% time)	10.0	27.0	<0.02
Fussing (% time)	0.1	16.0	<0.01
Crying (% time)	0.1	9.8	<0.02
Stress behavior (hiccupping; % time)	1.0	4.8	<0.01
Heart rate (beats/minute)	−6.5	0.7	<0.01
Vagal tone	0.3	0	<0.05

Criticisms and Limitations: The authors did not fully define outcomes (e.g., gross movement, infant weigh-in protocol) or fidelity procedures or report fidelity assessment outcomes. Both study conditions included a kinesthetic passive movement component, but the authors did not describe the reason for its inclusion in the intervention. Research suggests that infant race/ethnicity may impact access to quality NICUs and quality of care within the NICU (Horbar et al., 2019; Boghossian et al., 2019); however, the authors did not include demographic information about their sample or the NICU(s) where the study was conducted.

Other Relevant Studies and Information:

- Massage therapy, using either the Field et al. or another protocol, has consistently (although not always) yielded increases in weight gain in preterm infants in other studies, including multiple randomized controlled trials (Field et al., 1986; Ho et al., 2010; Mendes & Procianoy, 2008; Álvarez et al., 2017; Elmoneim et al., 2021). Other reported benefits include increases in natural killer cell cytotoxicity, brain development, bone mineralization, and motor performance as well as reductions in stress, length of hospital stay, and incidence of late-onset sepsis (Field et al., 1986; Ho et al., 2010; Mendes & Procianoy, 2008; Álvarez et al., 2017; Elmoneim et al., 2021).

- Field et al.'s work has shaped protocols utilized in NICU environments. For example, the Supporting and Enhancing NICU Sensory Experiences program, designed to facilitate parent-led, developmentally appropriate sensory experiences for high-risk infants in the NICU, incorporates infant massage as one of four possible tactile experiences (Pineda et al., 2019). This program, now implemented widely within the United States and abroad, has yielded improvements in both parental confidence and infant neurobehavioral performance (Pineda et al., 2020).

Summary and Implications: Preterm infants who received moderate-pressure massage therapy and kinesthetic stimulation gained more weight than those who received light-pressure massage therapy and kinesthetic stimulation. Further, findings suggest that the moderate-pressure massage therapy protocol was associated with less stress (i.e., hiccupping), more relaxed behavioral states (e.g., less active sleep, fussing, crying, less movement), and lower heart rate. Overall, the data indicate that providing moderate-pressure massage therapy and kinesthetic stimulation has the potential to improve outcomes for stable preterm infants.

CLINICAL CASE: MASSAGE THERAPY PROTOCOLS FOR PRETERM INFANTS IN THE NICU

Case History

Trevor, a preterm infant, was admitted to the NICU at 29 weeks' gestational age and currently weighs 1800 grams. His birth mother has given up her rights to care for the newborn, and his adoption paperwork has been finalized. The nurses have documented active sleep, clenched fists, tremors, and difficulty gaining weight in his chart. It is not uncommon to see him crying and fussing throughout the day. When his adoptive parents visit, they try to soothe him by gently touching his arms or legs, but they notice he becomes fussier. There have been no reports of maternal substance abuse during pregnancy, and no surgeries are anticipated. How can the occupational therapist working in the NICU environment contribute to multidisciplinary treatment planning when discussing this client?

Suggested Answer

Since Trevor presents with similar clinical symptoms as presented in this study, it may be beneficial to train members of the clinical team and/or his parents to implement a moderate-pressure massage therapy protocol in lieu of the light-touch tactile experiences currently provided by his parents. These light-touch experiences may be dysregulating and contributing to a higher arousal level, possibly resulting in increased energy expenditure and thereby negatively impacting weight gain. Sharing this study with the multidisciplinary team in the NICU may be beneficial to Trevor and other preterm infants.

References

Álvarez, M. J., Fernández, D., Gómez-Salgado, J., Rodríguez-González, D., Rosón, M., & Lapeña, S. (2017). The effects of massage therapy in hospitalized preterm neonates: A systematic review. *International Journal of Nursing Sciences, 69*, 119–136.

Boghossian, N. S., Geraci, M., Lorch, S. A., Phibbs, C. S., Edwards, E. M., & Horbar, J. D. (2019). Racial and ethnic differences over time in outcomes of infants born less than 30 weeks' gestation. *Pediatrics, 144*(3), Article e20191106.

Elmoneim, M. A., Mohamed, H. A., Awad, A., El-Hawary, A., Salem, N., El Helaly, R., Nasef, N., & Abdel-Hady, H. (2021). Effect of tactile/kinesthetic massage therapy on growth and body composition of preterm infants. *European Journal of Pediatrics, 180*, 207–215.

Field, T. M., Schanberg, S. M., Scafidi, F., Bauer, C. R., Vega-Lahr, N., Garcia, R., Nystrom, J., & Kuhn, C. M. (1986). Tactile/kinesthetic stimulation effects on preterm neonates. *Pediatrics, 77*(5), 654–658.

Ho, Y.-B., Lee, R. S. Y., Chow, C.-B., & Pang, M. Y. C. (2010). Impact of massage therapy on motor outcomes in very low-birthweight infants: Randomized controlled pilot study. *Pediatrics International, 52*, 378–385.

Horbar, J. D., Edwards, E. M., Greenberg, L. T., Profit, J., Draper, D., Helkey, D., Lorch, S. A., Lee, H. C., Phibbs, C. S., Rogowski, J., Gould, J. B., & Firebaugh, G. (2019). Racial segregation and inequality in the neonatal intensive care unit for very low-birth-weight and very preterm infants. *JAMA Pediatrics, 173*(5), 455–461.

Mendes, E. W., & Procianoy, R. S. (2008). Massage therapy reduces hospital stay and occurrence of late-onset sepsis in very preterm neonates. *Journal of Perinatology, 28*, 815–820.

Pineda, R., Raney, M., & Smith, J. (2019). Supporting and enhancing NICU sensory experiences (SENSE): Defining developmentally-appropriate sensory exposures for high-risk infants. *Early Human Development, 133*, 39–35.

Pineda, R., Wallendorf, M., & Smith, J. (2020). A pilot study demonstrating the impact of the supporting and enhancing NICU sensory experiences (SENSE) program on the mother and infant. *Early Human Development, 144*, 105000.

33

Exploring the Content Validity of the Pediatric Evaluation of Disability Inventory (PEDI)

Focusing on Functional Performance of Daily Living Activities

GUSTAVO REINOSO AND KAREN PARK

PEDI

> The results of the questionnaire provide the initial support for the content validity of the [Pediatric Disability Inventory]. In addition, the data indicate that the three measurement dimensions of the PEDI were found to be appropriate and consistent with providing a comprehensive description of function in children.
>
> HALEY, S. M., COSTER, W. J., & FAAS, R. M. (1991). *A content validity study of the Pediatric Evaluation of Disability Inventory. Pediatric Physical Therapy, 3(4),*
> *177–184.*

Original Paper: https://journals.lww.com/pedpt/Abstract/1991/00340/A_Content_Validity_Study_of_the_Pediatric.2.aspx

Research Question: Is the PEDI a valid and clinically feasible measure of a child's functional status?

Funding: US Department of Education, National Institute of Disability and Rehabilitation Research

Year Study Began: Not reported

Year Study Published: 1991

Study Location: Boston, MA

Who Was Studied: Experts in pediatric rehabilitation. Experts' average years of total experience in pediatric rehabilitation was 17.1 years (standard deviation [SD] = 7.4), and average years of clinical experience in pediatrics was 16.5 years (SD = 6.2); 70% had a terminal degree (PhD, ScD, MD), representing various clinical and academic roles (clinical practice, 23.2%; teaching, 33.8%; administration, 14.5%; and research, 26.5%). Nearly 90% were involved in some type of academic or clinical teaching role, and more than 80% had spent at least some percentage of time in a clinical practice role in pediatrics.

Who Was Excluded: Experts were ineligible for the panel if they were familiar with the test.

How Many Patients: 35 experts were selected to comprise the panel; 31 experts returned questionnaires

Study Overview: See Figure 33.1.

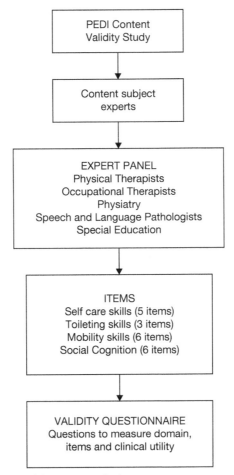

Figure 33.1. Overview of the PEDI study design.

Endpoints:

- PEDI items measure functional skills including self-care, mobility, and social function in children with disabilities.
- Comprehensiveness of PEDI items to assess pediatric functional skills.
- Adequacy of the three PEDI dimensions (functional skills, caregiver assistance with complex activities, and modifications).

RESULTS

- Eighty percent of experts judged the PEDI as either good or excellent on the two major content validity issues: 1) ability of the PEDI to measure functional disability in children and 2) ability of the PEDI to determine the comprehensiveness of the item sampling.
    - Eighty percent of experts judged the construct validity and comprehensiveness of three major domains (mobility, self-care, toileting) as good or excellent.
    - Seventy percent of experts judged the construct validity and comprehensiveness of the fourth domain (social cognition) as good or excellent.
- Eighty percent of experts gave either excellent or good ratings of the appropriateness of the three measurement scales (functional skills/behaviors, caregiver assistance, modifications) for the total PEDI, mobility domain, and toileting domain.
    - In the self-care domain, 78.6% of experts gave excellent or good ratings of the appropriateness of the measurement dimensions.
    - In the social function domain, 72.4% of experts gave excellent or good ratings of the appropriateness of the measurement dimensions.
- More than 80% of experts gave excellent or good ratings regarding the clinical meaningfulness of the description of functional status.
- Seventy-four percent of experts rated the overall PEDI as having good or excellent potential to detect clinically meaningful change.
    - In the self-care domain, 62.9% of experts rated the PEDI as having excellent or good potential to detect change.
    - In the social function domain, 48.4% of experts rated the PEDI as having excellent or good potential to detect change.
- More than 80% of experts rated the PEDI as a clinically feasible instrument when used as a parent report/structured interview or when administered by a therapist or educator.
- Forty-seven percent of experts indicated they would add more items to the PEDI
- Sixteen percent of experts indicated they would remove items from the PEDI.

Criticisms and Limitations:

- A few experts felt that the PEDI was potentially long and time-consuming, limiting its relevance for routine clinical use.
- The PEDI was felt to be a good measure of functional status but may not be appropriate to measure functional change, particularly in very young infants and children with more significant developmental delays in the social function domain.

Other Relevant Studies and Information:

- Following several years of research and clinical applications using the PEDI with populations, countries, and contexts, future directions were explored using item banks and adaptive testing (Haley et al., 2010).
- The PEDI was trialed using adaptive testing with excellent results. Discriminant validity showed ability to discriminate children with and without disabilities; test–retest reliability was excellent (intraclass correlation coefficient [ICC] = 0.96–0.99); and administration time was short (M = 12.66 minutes; SD = 4.47). Parents expressed positive reactions to administration using adaptive testing (Dumas et al., 2012).
- With a new way of administering the PEDI using computerized adaptive testing (CAT), a study examined the construct validity and test–retest reliability. A group (n = 101) of children with cerebral palsy were examined with the PEDI-CAT, and the Gross Motor Function Classification System level and convergent and divergent validity were explored. Results demonstrated robust construct validity and high test–retest reliability (ICC = 0.96–0.99) (Shore et al., 2019).

Summary and Implications: The PEDI tool for assessing disability in children covers domains in self-care, mobility, toileting, and social cognition and captures functional skills, caregiver assistance, and environmental modifications. In this analysis, an expert panel found the tool to be a valid and clinically feasible measure of a child's functional status.

CLINICAL CASE: EVALUATING PARTICIPATION WITH THE PEDI

Case History

Valentina, a Hispanic 5-year-old child with a diagnosis of spastic cerebral palsy, was referred for an occupational therapy assessment. Her mother wanted a more accurate picture of how to promote Valentina's participation during self-care (e.g., eating and dressing) and mobility (transfers to and from her manual wheelchair). She expressed that Valentina's teacher and aide believe she performs more independently and with less assistance at school versus in the home environment. Her mother also reported that, at times, she feels she helps Valentina more than she should.

Suggested Answer

The occupational therapist completed the PEDI-CAT to assess Valentina's level of ability to successfully participate in activities of daily living and mobility tasks. The outcomes reported on daily activities, mobility, social cognition, and responsibility indicated that Valentina was more independent in the school setting. For example, it was reported that she was able to feed herself using a fork and spoon at school. A discussion with Valentina's caregivers allowed mom to lessen her support around feeding. The occupational therapist and family discussed strategies to provide more opportunities to engage in self-feeding in the home. Additionally, Valentina's mother requested to meet more regularly with all individuals providing services and interacting with Valentina to develop more appropriate goals across different settings.

References

Dumas, H. M., Fragala-Pinkham, M. A., Haley, S. M., Ni, P., Coster, W., Kramer, J. M., Kao, Y. C., Moed, R., & Ludlow, L. H. (2012). Computer adaptive test performance in children with and without disabilities: Prospective field study of the PEDI-CAT. *Disability and Rehabilitation, 34*(5), 393–401. https://doi.org/10.3109/09638 288.2011.607217

Haley, S. M., Coster, W. I., Kao, Y. C., Dumas, H. M., Fragala-Pinkham, M. A., Kramer, J. M., Ludlow, L. H., & Moed, R. (2010). Lessons from use of the Pediatric Evaluation of Disability Inventory: Where do we go from here? *Pediatric Physical Therapy: The Official Publication of the Section on Pediatrics of the American Physical Therapy Association, 22*(1), 69–75. https://doi.org/10.1097/PEP.0b013e3181cbfbf6

Shore, B. J., Allar, B. G., Miller, P. E., Matheney, T. H., Snyder, B. D., & Fragala-Pinkham, M. (2019). Measuring the reliability and construct validity of the Pediatric Evaluation of Disability Inventory-Computer Adaptive Test (PEDI-CAT) in children with cerebral palsy. *Archives of Physical Medicine and Rehabilitation, 100*(1), 45–51. https://doi. org/10.1016/j.apmr.2018.07.427

34

Evaluating Playfulness in Children

KARLA K. AUSDERAU AND CANDACE CHATMAN

While our results must be viewed with caution [as participant data rated at 92% instead of 95% fit to the Rasch model], we also found that the mean ToP score of children with physical disabilities did not differ from that of their able-bodied peers.

HARKNESS, L., & BUNDY, A. (2001). The test of playfulness and children with physical disabilities. *The Occupational Therapy Journal of Research*, 21(2), 73–89.

Original Paper: https://doi.org/10.1177/153944920102100203

Research Question:

1. Is the Test of Playfulness (ToP), an assessment instrument originally validated with children without disabilities, reliable and valid for children with physical disabilities and no known cognitive limitations?
2. How do ToP scores and differences in test item patterns compare between children with physical disabilities and able-bodied peers?

Funding: None reported.

Year Study Began: Extant ToP normative data set collected in 1998

Year Study Published: 2001

Study Location: Colorado; Massachusetts; South Carolina; Ontario, Canada

Who Was Studied: Twenty-five children (2–12 years old) with no known physical disabilities or cognitive limitations from the ToP normative data set (Bundy, 2001) and 25 children with physical disabilities without cognitive disabilities matched by gender and age.

Who Was Excluded: Children with known cognitive limitations. Children who were part of the normative data set for the ToP who were not matched with the 25 children with physical disabilities.

How Many Patients: 50

Study Overview: See Figure 34.1.

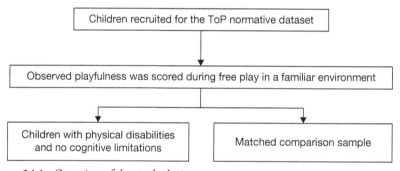

Figure 34.1. Overview of the study design.

Study Intervention: Children's playfulness was rated using the ToP, a standardized assessment for children from 6 months of age that measures play across four elements (intrinsic motivation, suspension of reality, internal control, and framing) using 29 items scored on a 4-point Likert scale. Two 15-minute free-play sessions in familiar environments with the majority occurring in both indoor and outdoor settings were videotaped. Examiners did not interact with the children unless there was a safety concern. Each video was scored by a minimum of two trained reliable raters.

Endpoints:

- Primary outcomes: Reliability and validity of the ToP as demonstrated by goodness of fit of the data to the Rasch measurement model.
- Secondary outcomes: Patterns of playfulness in ToP test items and ToP mean scores.

RESULTS

- Rater reliability was confirmed with 100% of study raters conforming to expectations of the Rasch model.
- Regarding person-response validity (valid for children with disabilities), 88% of children with physical disabilities ($n = 22$) fit within the acceptable range of the fit statistics but fell below the identified 95% fit standard. The <95% model fit suggests that the ToP results from children with physical disabilities in this study did not conform to the same model created with children without physical disabilities, indicating that a different hierarchy of difficulty of test items may be required to appropriately describe playfulness in children with physical disabilities.
- Seventy-two percent ($n = 18$) of children with physical disabilities received at least one unexpected score on the 24 items of the ToP—scoring either poorly on an easy item or highly on a more difficult item.
- Four ToP items that had unexpected ratings (low scores on easy items or high scores on difficult items) for at least six children (24%) with physical disabilities were *decides* (unexpectedly low), *process* (unexpectedly low), *exuberance* (unexpectedly high), and *clowns/jokes* (unexpectedly high). Unexpected ratings on ToP items require further investigation with a larger sample to clarify the meaning.
- Mean ToP scores between the two groups did not differ significantly; 19 of the 25 children with physical disabilities scored above the mean for the entire sample of children without disabilities in the normative sample.

Criticism and Limitations: The small sample limited the ability to find patterns in item differences or determine how varying physical disabilities or mobility levels influence ToP performance. The environment where free play occurred was not controlled, which may have influenced level of challenge, familiarity, and physical opportunities for either group.

Other Relevant Studies and Information:

- Bundy et al. (2001) focused on the original development and psychometric properties of the ToP primarily with children without special needs (92%, $n = 197$). The authors found the ToP to be a valid (construct and concurrent) and reliable (interrater) assessment to evaluate playfulness in children.
- The Test of Environmental Supports (TOES) was developed for concurrent use with ToP to assess the supportiveness of the play

environment and environmental influence on child's playfulness. The TOES was found to have good interrater reliability but was not sensitive to child–environment fit (Bronson & Bundy, 2001).
- The ToP was used to assess playfulness in children with cerebral palsy; higher gross motor functioning and adaptive behavior were both associated with increased playfulness (Chiarello et al., 2019). Gross motor skills and adaptive behavior may support playfulness in children with cerebral palsy.

Summary and Implications: Based on the results from this study, the ToP is a reliable assessment of playfulness for children with physical disabilities as mean ToP scores did not differ between children with physical disabilities and those without. However, person-response validity was not established, and it is yet to be determined if it is necessary to create a ToP data set specifically for children with physical disabilities. Further investigation is needed to determine if the ToP is a valid assessment for children with physical disabilities and how the environment influences playfulness for children with or without disabilities.

CLINICAL CASE: PLAYFULNESS IN CHILDREN WITH CEREBRAL PALSY

Case History
Kai, a 5-year-old boy with spastic cerebral palsy and no identified cognitive limitations, was referred for an occupational therapy evaluation to assess the his occupational performance in school and frequented community contexts. Specifically, Kai's family is concerned about how their son is engaging in play behaviors that may support peer engagement and participation in age-appropriate activities.

Suggested Answer
The ToP has preliminary evidence to support its use as an assessment tool for children ages 2–12 years with physical disabilities in familiar environments with familiar peers, which would be appropriate for the child referred and would address the family's concerns. The occupational therapist can be confident in the reliability of the ToP but should be cautious when comparing Kai's results with the playfulness patterns of other children. In addition, when evaluating the child's play, he should be observed in an environment that allows him to physically negotiate the space.

References

Bronson, M. R., & Bundy, A. C. (2001). A correlational study of a test of playfulness and a test of environmental supportiveness for play. *The Occupational Therapy Journal of Research, 21*(4), 241–259. https://doi.org/10.1177/153944920102100403

Bundy, A., Nelson, L., Metzger, M., & Bingaman, K. (2001). Validity and reliability of a test of playfulness. *The Occupational Therapy Journal of Research, 21*(4), 276–292. https://doi.org/10.1177/153944920102100405

Chiarello, L. A., Bartlett, D. J., Palisano, R. J., McCoy, S. W., Jeffries, L., Fiss, A. L., & Wilk, P. (2019). Determinants of playfulness of young children with cerebral palsy. *Developmental Neurorehabilitation, 22*(4), 240–249. https://doi.org/10.1080/17518 423.2018.1471623

35

Environmental Barriers and Their Impact on Participation for Youth with Physical Disabilities

KARRIE KINGSLEY AND TARA J. GLENNON

The highest overall impact of barriers was associated with school and work followed by the physical and structural environment and policies.... Because children spend so much time in school it is not surprising that barriers, when present, are perceived by parents as having a significant impact.

LAW, M., PETRENCHIK, T., KING, G., & HURLEY, P. (2007). Perceived environmental barriers to recreational, community, and school participation for children and youth with physical disabilities. *Archives of Physical Medicine and Rehabilitation*, 88(12), 1636–1942.

Original Paper: https://doi.org/10.1016/j.apmr.2007.07.035

Research Question: What are the perceived environmental barriers to recreational, community, and school participation for a large group of school-age children with a range of health conditions and disabilities?

Funding: National Institutes of Health, the CanChild Centre for Childhood Disability Research, the Ontario Ministry of Health and Longterm Care, the Research Alliance for Children with Special Needs, and the Social Sciences and Research Council of Canada

Year Study Began: 2001

Year Study Published: 2007

Study Location: Province of Ontario, Canada, within 11 publicly funded children's rehabilitation centers and a children's hospital.

Who Was Studied: Parents and children with a range of health and developmental problems, including 51% diagnosed with cerebral palsy, nearly one-third demonstrating significant behavioral problems (score of 17 or above on the Strengths and Difficulties Questionnaire and a mean summary score of 70.3% on the Activity Scale for Kids).

Who Was Excluded: This was a random selection of a cross-sectional sample with no exclusion criteria.

How Many Patients: 427 parent–child pairs

Study Overview: Non-experimental design utilizing a secondary analysis of initial cross-sectional data from a longitudinal study (Figure 35.1). Data collection included initial questionnaires/measures of health, family cohesion, social supports, and child's behavioral health status completed by the primary caregiver; a home visit and interview with self-identified person who was knowledgeable about the child's daily activities; parent-reported perceptions of environmental barriers; and child self-assessment of functional status, activity preferences, and measures of recreational/leisure participation. Data regarding perception of barriers were analyzed by age group, behavior, and physical functioning.

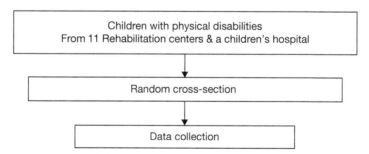

Figure 35.1. Overview of the study design.

Endpoints:

- Perceived environmental barriers, as measured by the Craig Hospital Inventory of Environmental Factors (CHIEF)

RESULTS

- The study sample included 229 boys and 198 girls in three age cohorts (6–8, 9–11, 12–14 years) with the majority (41%) at 9–11 years.
- Based on caregiver reports utilizing the CHIEF, perceived barriers were ranked highest to lowest in school and work, natural and built environments, policies, services and assistance, and attitudes, respectively.
- Multivariate analysis of covariance results yielded significant main effects for age of the children, level of physical functioning, and degree of behavioral problems:
  - For the mean impact of barriers, children in the 12–14 year range experienced higher impact than the 9–11 and 6–8 year cohorts.
  - Children with lower physical functioning (<25th percentile on the Activity Scale for Kids) experienced significantly greater impact of barriers in the contexts of service and assistance, school and work, and policies, as well as significantly greater barriers in the natural and built environment context.
  - Children with significant behavioral problems (≥17 [upper range of cutoff scores to minimize false positives] on the Strengths and Difficulties Questionnaire) experienced a higher impact of barriers in all contexts.
- The intersection of younger age and lower physical functioning led to increased experience of barriers in all five contexts (Table 35.1).

TABLE 35.1. MEAN MAGNITUDE OF REPORTED BARRIERS TO
PARTICIPATION BY ASK PERCENTILE GROUPS

CHIEF Subscale	Mean Magnitude	ASK <25th $p < 0.01$	ASK 25th–50th $p < 0.01$	ASK 50th–75th $p < 0.01$	ASK >75th $p < 0.01$	SDQ $p < 0.01$ No Behavioral Problems	SDQ $p < 0.01$ Behavioral Problems
Services and assistance	1.02 ± 1.20	1.70	1.06	0.85	0.47	0.95	1.22
Attitudes	0.88 ± 1.18	0.86	1.00	1.02	0.62	0.69	1.37
School and work	1.55 ± 1.88	1.89	1.46	1.75	1.10	1.26	2.32
Natural and built environments	1.31 ± 1.35	2.07	1.53	1.02	0.59	1.30	1.34
Policies	1.24 ± 1.71	1.84	1.33	1.23	0.55	1.10	1.61

ASK = Activity Scale for Kids; SDQ = Strengths and Difficulties Questionnaire.

Criticisms and Limitations: The CHIEF is not validated on children with disabilities, and all data were from self-reports and parent perception. The parent sample was comprised of 91% White, 89% mothers, and 83% from two-parent families with incomes above the median, limiting the generalizability of the outcomes to other communities or single-parent households.

Other Relevant Studies and Information:

- Domain-specific participation was noted to be decreased in young children (36–72 months) with cerebral palsy compared to typically developing children, with community mobility the most impacted and the domestic domain the least impacted (Abu-Dahab et al., 2020). Parent perceptions (e.g., of the child's ability or of the environmental supports available) contributed to the child's level of participation.
- Children who were less impaired, and thus able to have more frequent participation, demonstrated a higher quality of life (Williams et al., 2021).
- The primary elements of meaningful participation are enjoyment (memorable and exciting, comfortable physical sensations), capability (e.g., the experience of succeeding; surpassing oneself in activities that called for courage, skills, knowledge; or attentional ability to do the same activity as others), social involvement (e.g., doing the same activity as others, belonging to a specific group), and autonomy (e.g., making choices and decisions). Children have a curiosity to learn and develop their abilities and want to be actively making choices and creating solutions which enable them to engage in a preferred activity (Vänskä et al., 2020).
- The World Health Organization's (WHO's; 2001) definition of impairment versus disability (e.g., barriers and attitudes that disable individuals) led to the understanding that the strategies required to improve participation should come from a social, cultural, and community perspective. Understanding the barriers to participation, as well as the WHO's perspective, helped shape the 2010 American with Disabilities Act's standards for accessible design (US Department of Justice, 2010) for new construction and alterations, school-based initiatives for more inclusive practices, and an overall commitment to provide better access for persons with an impairment.

Summary and Implications: Parents of children with health and developmental challenges perceive barriers across multiple contexts, which limit their child's participation in recreational, school, and community activities. School barriers, such as bullying, social marginalization, and fiscal challenges, had the most impact. While encouraging community attitudes were noted, they did not appear to translate into substantive policy or structural changes. As adolescents attempt to expand recreational and leisure participation outside of home and school and into the community, perceived environmental barriers increase. Children and youth with behavioral challenges were perceived to have significantly greater barriers other than those of the physical environment.

CLINICAL CASE: GREATER INDEPENDENCE AND PARTICIPATION IN SCHOOL

Case History

The school-based occupational therapy practitioner (OTP) received a referral for Madison (they/them), a 14-year-old high school student diagnosed with cerebral palsy and increased spasticity in the arms. Through the occupational profile, both Madison and teaching staff noted concerns with independently accessing the various locations within the school campus, as well as mobility of their communication device when out of the classroom. After asking Madison several questions related to access and participation across school and other environments, the OTP and Madison concluded that their participation with peers when not accompanied by an adult was compromised, as was communication with peers during school-related recreational and social situations. Based on the occupational therapy assessment, Madison was a Level IV on the Gross Motor Function Classification System (Russell et al., 2002).

Suggested Answer

Based on the OTP's familiarity of Law et al.'s findings, the OTP appreciated that adolescents are expanding their recreational and leisure pursuits, as well as independence from adults. When considering Madison's age and gross motor functioning level, the OTP discussed with the team the potential impact of these barriers to greater independence. Thereafter, the OTP shared Madison's participation preferences that were identified during the evaluation process. During the individualized education program meeting, the OTP made several recommendations based on Madison's perceptions of barriers, thus improving opportunities for independently navigating the built environment at school; presented options to secure the communication device to the motorized wheelchair; and highlighted the need for a team-based program to support Madison's ability to advocate for their participation in school-based extracurricular programs.

References

Abu-Dahab, S. M. N., Alheresh, R. A., Malkawi, S. H., Saleh, M., & Wong, J. (2020). Participation patterns and determinants of participation of young children with cerebral palsy. *Australian Occupational Therapy Journal, 68*(3), 195–204. https://doi.org/10.1111/1440-1630.12714

Russell, D. J., Rosenbaum, P. L., Avery, L., & Lane, M. (2002). *Gross motor function measure (GMFM-66 and GMFM-88) user's manual: Clinics in developmental medicine.* Mac Keith Press.

US Department of Justice. (2010). *ADA standards for accessible design.*

Vänskä, N., Sipari, S., & Haataja, L. (2020). What makes participation meaningful? Using photo-elicitation to interview children with disabilities. *Physical & Occupational Therapy in Pediatrics, 40*(6), 595–609. https://doi.org/10.1080/01942638.2020.1736234

Williams, K., Jacoby, P., Whitehouse, A., Kim, R., Epstein, A., Murphy, N., Reid, S., Leonard, H., Reddinhough, D., & Down, J. (2021). Functioning, participation, and quality of life in children with intellectual disability: An observational study. *Developmental Medicine & Child Neurology, 63*, 89–96.

World Health Organization. (2001). *International classification of functioning, disability and health.*

36

The Importance of Family-Centered Care

DOMINIQUE H. COMO AND STEFANIE BODISON

In this article, we present a number of critical dilemmas that are based on data drawn from ethnographic research, descriptive studies, and training seminars we conducted with pediatric practitioners and parents of children with special health care needs. These dilemmas highlight the complexities involved in building effective partnerships among all the key players, the influence of multiple cultural worlds on everyday practices, and the need to provide supports to practitioners for the emotional and social dimensions of practice.

LAWLOR, M. C., & MATTINGLY, C. F. (1997). The complexities embedded in family-centered care. *American Journal of Occupational Therapy, 52*(4), 259–267.

Original Paper: https://doi.org/10.5014/ajot.52.4.259

Research Question: How do healthcare practitioners most effectively involve family in the pediatric care of children with special healthcare needs, and what are the roadblocks in doing so?

Funding: The Maternal and Child Health Division, Department of Health and Human Services; the Early Education Program for Children with Disabilities, Office of Special Education Programs; the Office of Special Education and Rehabilitation Services, Department of Education; and the American Occupational Therapy Foundation

Year Study Began:

- Study 1: 1987
- Study 2: 1990
- Study 3: 1990

Year Study Published: 1997

Study Location: Chicago, IL; Los Angeles, CA

Who Was Studied: Families (mothers) of children with special healthcare needs or in special education programs, healthcare practitioners, and special education professionals.

Who Was Excluded: Not applicable

How Many Participants:

- Study 1: Unknown
- Study 2: 20
- Study 3: 27

Study Overview: This article is a critique of traditional, clinician-focused models of intervention, based on data from three qualitative studies focused on family-centered care, that addresses the challenges, or "daily dilemmas," that arise when attempting to create family–practitioner partnerships (Figure 36.1).

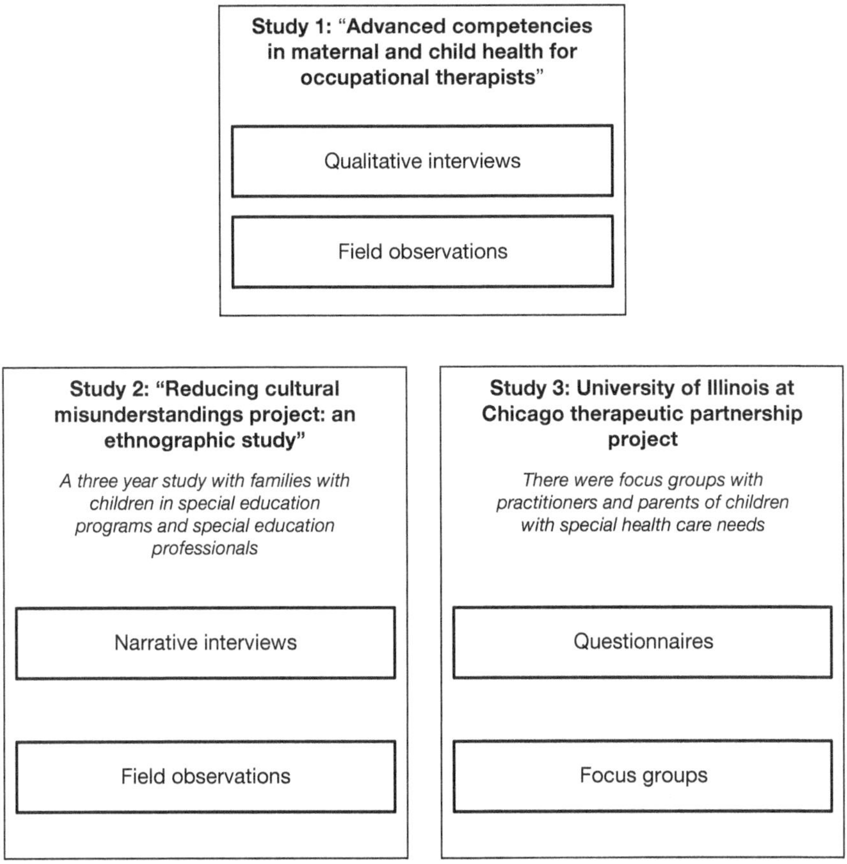

Study 1: "Advanced competencies in maternal and child health for occupational therapists"

Qualitative interviews

Field observations

Study 2: "Reducing cultural misunderstandings project: an ethnographic study"

A three year study with families with children in special education programs and special education professionals

Narrative interviews

Field observations

Study 3: University of Illinois at Chicago therapeutic partnership project

There were focus groups with practitioners and parents of children with special health care needs

Questionnaires

Focus groups

Figure 36.1. Overview of the study design.

Study Intervention: Not applicable

RESULTS

Lawlor and Mattingly identified two critiques to adapting family-centered care:

Situating Family-Centered Care in Cultural Contexts is defined as the clinic culture in which healthcare practices are immersed and which shapes the understanding of practitioners' actions, their communication, and the nature of their work. Three themes emerged from the data related to this category:

- Professional as Expert
  - An expert model of treatment is often the default in healthcare settings. In this model, the professional–client relationship is hierarchical, and the client's role is limited to simply providing information to the expert,

then complying with the intervention plan as prescribed. Often, the power and control reside with the practitioner. Under this model, even when attempts are made to include the client/family, it is limited to attaining "buy-in" to the professional's plan.

- The Nature of "Real Work"
  - o The research highlighted that practitioners often divided their work into "real treatment" and rapport-building (e.g., "chitchat," "making the patient comfortable"). Real treatment was described as that which could be noted in charts, discussed in staff meetings, and reported to insurance agencies—often seen as more legitimate. Practitioners expressed concerns about meeting professional responsibilities while also delivering care that meets the concerns of the family. Typical clinic culture often favors the actions associated with "real treatment" over the oft unbillable, soft skills associated with building rapport.
- Service Fragmentation and Specialization
  - o Clinic culture also influences the way collaborative work can occur. At times, "turf battles" can develop as professionals attempt to maintain their autonomy. This can be exacerbated when needs identified by clients do not align with the specialized services, highlighting gaps in the service network. Additionally, different professionals may identify the same problem in different ways, thereby seeing the child, the disability, and the intervention from different lenses, making collaboration challenging.

Daily Dilemmas within Family-Centered Care identified challenges to effectively develop family–practitioner partnerships. Two themes emerged from the data related to this category:

- Practitioner Dilemmas
  - o Working with the family means that it is not often clear who the client actually is, and some practitioners find that expanding their care to the family often means that clear delineation of the problem begins to blur, making them question their effectiveness. Furthermore, professional boundaries are tested as practitioners are often tasked with addressing patient–family concerns that rarely align with practitioner specializations.
  - o Practitioners also described having difficulty navigating collaborations with families that did not share their cultural backgrounds, with families that did not resemble "traditional" configurations, and with

families where the professional boundaries began to erode (e.g., "just like family," "friend") or the emotional/social needs seemed too great.

- Family Dilemmas
  o Families described their own challenges developing effective collaborations with practitioners, including feeling judged by practitioners as they insert themselves into the service delivery process, not always feeling like implicit social contracts were being met (e.g., failing to call, keeping parent waiting, not being clear about what practitioner is thinking), and feeling like they were operating on a different timeframe than the practitioners (practitioners focus on short-term goals vs. families' interest in long-term goals). Families also highlighted the need for practitioners to like their child (e.g., value the child, enjoy the child, engage the child), with mothers often identified as cultural brokers who aid in this process by attending appointments and meetings, serving as the family representative.

Criticisms and Limitations: The analysis of the data is based on three studies which had primary goals not specifically focused on family-centered care. Different insights may have emerged from a study that was specifically focused on family-centered care.

Other Relevant Studies and Information:

- A 2018 meta-analysis analyzed 15 studies that used the Measure of Processes of Care (MPOC) to evaluate parent perception of family-centered care for their rehabilitation (Almasri et al., 2018). Of the five MPOC subscales, *Enabling & Partnership, Providing Specific Information about the Child, Coordinated & Comprehensive Care,* and *Respectful & Supportive Care* received aggregated mean scores ranging from 5.0 to 5.5, indicating that on average parents thought these practices were provided to a "fairly great extent." However, *Providing General Information* received the lowest aggregated mean scores, requiring more attention, which was highlighted by the qualitative studies which indicated that opportunities for communication with providers were desired.
- In 2012, the American Academy of Pediatrics published a policy statement that emphasized that patient-centered care and family-centered care were core principles, outcomes, and key benefits of any healthcare services provided. They noted that family-centered care is

associated with significant reduction of anxiety for children and parents, improves staff satisfaction, and decreases healthcare costs, among many other benefits (Committee on Hospital Care & Institute for Patient- and Family-Centered Care, 2012).

• Lawlor & Mattingly have published numerous works stemming from their longitudinal ethnographic studies, which highlight the use of narrative stories to help researchers and healthcare professionals understand those who may face power imbalance in the healthcare system and the "work" that underserved, specifically African American, mothers must undertake to make their stories heard and understood by others, including healthcare professionals (Jacobs et al., 2011; Mattingly & Lawlor, 2000).

Summary and Implications: High-quality, effective, family-centered care offers many benefits for the child and family; but it is not accomplished without first addressing the "daily dilemmas" that might impede the development of a family–practitioner partnership. Practitioners often have to overcome the "traditional" clinical culture that places them in an expert position, reinforcing imbalanced power dynamics, while also preparing to address a wide array of concerns. To be implemented successfully, effective family-centered care requires a radical shift in human services.

CLINICAL CASE: CREATING EFFECTIVE PARTNERSHIPS WITH FAMILIES WHILE BEING MINDFUL OF POWER DYNAMICS

Case History

Jeremiah, an African American child with complex healthcare needs, is part of a non-traditional family and requires in-home therapy services because he is too medically fragile to leave his home. The therapist working with him provides services weekly and is focused on training his moms on the ways they can support the development of his feeding and eating skills. Based on Lawlor and Mattingly's findings, what should the therapist take into consideration in order to create an effective partnership with the family?

Suggested Answer

The occupational therapist is consciously aware of the imbalanced power dynamics that have the potential to situate her as the expert and the only one capable of improving Jeremiah's feeding and eating abilities. By consciously working to empower his caregivers and supporting their developing strengths through her words and actions (i.e., collaborating with family to develop goals, abiding by implicit social constructs, holding monthly meetings with other service providers, and displaying cultural humility), the occupational therapist is attempting to shift the way healthcare services are provided.

References

Almasri, N. A., An, M., & Palisano, R. J. (2018). Parents' perception of receiving family-centered care for their children with physical disabilities: A meta-analysis. *Physical & Occupational Therapy in Pediatrics, 38*(4), 427–443. https://doi.org/10.1080/01942 638.2017.1337664

Committee on Hospital Care & Institute for Patient- and Family-Centered Care. (2012). Patient- and family-centered care and the pediatrician's role. *Pediatrics, 129*(2), 394–404. https://doi.org/10.1542/peds.2011-3084

Jacobs, L., Lawlor, M., & Mattingly, C. (2011). I/we narratives among African American families raising children with special needs. *Culture, Medicine, and Psychiatry, 35*(1), 3–25. https://doi.org/10.1007/s11013-010-9196-5

Mattingly, C., & Lawlor, M. (2000). Learning from stories: Narrative interviewing in cross-cultural research. *Scandinavian Journal of Occupational Therapy, 7*(1), 4–14. https://doi.org/10.1080/110381200443571

Effectiveness of Occupational Therapy for Children with Sensory Modulation Disorder

STACEY REYNOLDS AND KAELAH POU

The findings suggest that OT-SI may be effective in ameliorating difficulties of children with [sensory modulation disorder].

MILLER, L. J., COLL, J. R., & SCHOEN, S. A. (2007). A randomized controlled pilot study of the effectiveness of occupational therapy for children with sensory modulation disorder. *American Journal of Occupational Therapy*, 61(2), 228–238.

Original Paper: https://pubmed.ncbi.nlm.nih.gov/17436845/

Research Question: Does occupational therapy using a sensory integration approach (OT-SI) improve attention, cognitive/social, sensory, or behavioral problems more than an active alternate placebo treatment (Activity Protocol) or a passive placebo (e.g., no treatment) for children with SMD?

Funding: The National Institutes of Health, the Wallace Foundation, and the American Occupational Therapy Foundation. Additional support provided by The Children's Hospital of Denver and the Coleman Institute for Cognitive Disabilities.

Year Study Began: 2001

Year Study Published: 2007

Study Location: Denver, CO

Who Was Studied: Children between the ages of 3 and 11.6 years with a clinical diagnosis of SMD referred to outpatient OT at The Children's Hospital of Denver.

- 25% female, 75% male
- 91.6% Caucasian, 4.2% Hispanic, 4.2% other
- Mean age = 6.58 years

Who Was Excluded:

- Children with IQ <85
- Children having received previous OT (not including school-based OT)
- Children with other diagnostic conditions (except for attention deficit hyperactivity disorder [ADHD], learning disabilities, or anxiety symptoms)
- Children enrolled in special education services resulting in pull-out services

How Many Patients: 24

Study Overview: Study participants were randomized to one of three groups: OT-SI, Activity Protocol, and no treatment (Figure 37.1).

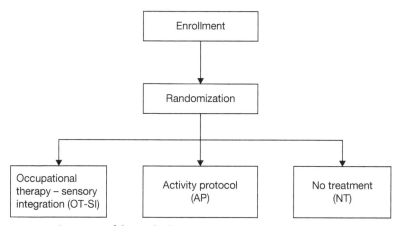

Figure 37.1. Overview of the study design.

Study Intervention: Children in the experimental group (OT-SI) group received treatment twice per week for 10 weeks. Sessions followed a manualized protocol based on sensory integration theory (Ayres, 1972), and a fidelity-to-treatment measure was used. Sessions took place in a large OT room equipped with sensory activities and toys; the therapist guided and scaffolded the child's participation in the sessions, and parents participated actively guided by the therapist. During sessions children interacted with sensory materials in an "active, meaningful, and fun manner" (p. 231).

Children in the alternative placebo group, otherwise known as the Activity Protocol group, participated in tabletop activities such as puzzles, arts and crafts, blocks, reading stories, and playing interactive games two times per week for 10 weeks. Activities were supported by non-OT staff members or graduate students who had education or psychology degrees and experience with young children. Sessions took place in the same-size room as the OT-SI sessions. Parent education and coaching was not a part of the Activity Protocol.

Children in the no-treatment group were placed on a 10-week wait list for OT-SI.

Follow-Up: Participants were tested pre-intervention (Week 1) and post-intervention (Week 11).

Endpoints:

Primary outcomes:

- Attention and Cognitive/Social Skills (Leiter International Performance Scale-Revised: Parent Rating Scale [Leiter-R])
- Behaviors related to Sensory Responsivity (Short Sensory Profile)
- Functional socialization skills (Vineland Adaptive Behavior Scales—Socialization Subtest)
- Internalizing and Externalizing behaviors (Child Behavior Checklist)
- Individualized Functional Goals (Goal Attainment Scaling)
- Electrodermal Reactivity (skin conductance during a sensory challenge protocol)

RESULTS

- Children in the OT-SI group made significantly greater gains in Goal Attainment Scaling compared to children in the Activity Protocol group ($p < 0.0001$) and the no-treatment group ($p < 0.0001$)

- Children in the OT-SI group made significantly greater improvements on the Attention domain of the Leiter-R compared to the no-treatment group ($p = 0.03$)
- Children in the OT-SI group made significantly greater improvements on the Cognitive/Social domain of the Leiter-R compared to the Activity Protocol group ($p = 0.02$)
- Children in the OT-SI group showed greater reduction in amplitudes of electrodermal responses compared to the Activity Protocol and no-treatment groups; however, this finding was not statistically significant.
- Children in the Activity Protocol group made greater but non-significant ($p = 0.49$) gains compared to the OT-SI group and no-treatment group on the Socialization subtest of the Vineland.
- Effect sizes were as follows: Leiter-R Attention and Cognitive/Social (0.29), Short Sensory Profile total score (0.08), Vineland Socialization subtest (0.14), Child Behavior Checklist Externalizing (0.10), Child Behavior Checklist Internalizing (0.07), and Goal Attainment Scaling (1.62).

Criticisms and Limitations: This study is limited by a small sample size and lack of statistical power, limiting both internal and external validity. Results may not generalize to those children who have low IQ or are receiving special education services.

Other Relevant Studies and Information:

- A systematic review by Schaaf and colleagues (2018) suggested that there is strong evidence for the use of Ayres Sensory Integration (also known as OT-SI) for improving individually generated goals of functioning and participation as measured by Goal Attainment Scaling for children with autism and challenges in processing and integrating sensory information.
- Similar gains in functional goal attainment have been demonstrated in children with sensory-based motor disorders using the OT-SI approach (Andelin et al., 2021).
- A fidelity measure has been developed and validated for use in research on Ayres Sensory Integration (also known as OT-SI) (May-Benson et al., 2014; Parham et al., 2011).

Summary and Implications: OT-SI had favorable effects on individual goal attainment, attention, and cognitive/social domains among children with SMD.

This treatment is recommended for such children when deficits in sensory processing and integration interfere with participation in meaningful activities or occupational performance. This study also provided a framework for future clinical trials (e.g., use of a manualized approach and fidelity measure) and identified outcome measures that were both meaningful and sensitive to change.

CLINICAL CASE: OT FOR CHILDREN WITH SENSORY MODULATION CHALLENGES

Case History

Angus (he/him), a 7-year-old boy, recently adopted, is referred for an outpatient OT evaluation due to parent and teacher concerns of poor attention, high levels of anxiety, lack of friends, and behaviors consistent with SMD (hyperreactivity type). He was evaluated by a psychiatrist and placed on medication to treat ADHD. Despite this intervention, Angus is continuing to have difficulty functioning in home, school, and community settings. Client and family goals focus mostly on Angus being able to participate in family and peer activities (e.g., birthday parties, cookouts) and to complete self-care tasks independently at school (e.g., flush the toilet in the public bathroom, participate in school assembly). As the treating occupational therapist, based on the results of this study, what type of intervention approach is indicated?

Suggested Answer

This study found that OT-SI is effective for improving individual functional goals as well as aspects of attention and social functioning in children with SMD. The child in this vignette presents with many signs of SMD as well as behaviors often associated with SMD hyperreactivity type such as anxiety and poor attention. Many of the children enrolled in the study also had comorbid ADHD, which is present in this client as well. Use of the OT-SI approach over a period of 10 weeks (two sessions per week) is recommended to support amelioration of sensory-based behaviors and enhance his ability to participate across environments. In accordance with the OT-SI approach, intervention activities should be performed within the context of play and encourage active involvement of the child in both planning and execution of the activity. During sessions, the therapist will serve to facilitate adaptive responses and present the "just right challenge" during sensorimotor tasks. Given that this child was recently adopted, the OT-SI approach may also be selected over other intervention approaches given its inclusion of parental coaching, education, and active participation.

References

Andelin, L., Schoen, S., & Reynolds, S. (2021). Effectiveness of occupational therapy using a sensory integration approach: A multiple baseline design study. *American Journal of Occupational Therapy, 75*(6), 76–85.

Ayres, A. J. (1972). *Sensory integration and learning disorders.* Western Psychological Services.

May-Benson, T. A., Roley, S. S., Mailloux, Z., Parham, L. D., Koomar, J., Schaaf, R. C., Jaarsveld, A. V., & Cohn, E. (2014). Interrater reliability and discriminative validity of the structural elements of the Ayres Sensory Integration Fidelity Measure. *American Journal of Occupational Therapy, 68*(5), 506–513. https://doi.org/10.5014/ajot.2014.010652

Parham, L. D., Roley, S. S., May-Benson, T. A., Koomar, J., Brett-Green, B., Burke, J. P., Cohn, E. S., Mailloux, Z., Miller, L. J., & Schaaf, R. C. (2011). Development of a fidelity measure for research on the effectiveness of the Ayres Sensory Integration° intervention. *American Journal of Occupational Therapy, 65*(2), 133–142. https://doi.org/10.5014/ajot.2011.000745

Schaaf, R. C., Dumont, R. L., Arbesman, M., & May-Benson, T. A. (2018). Efficacy of occupational therapy using Ayres Sensory Integration°: A systematic review. *American Journal of Occupational Therapy, 72*(1), 7201190010p1–7201190010p10. https://doi.org/10.5014/ajot.2018.028431

SECTION 6

Rehabilitation and Disability

The intentional and strategic use of *occupation* as both a means and ends of occupational therapy (OT) intervention are what make OT distinctly valuable, effective, and patient-driven (Gray, 1998). In the physical rehabilitation setting, the OT evaluation reveals the patient's strengths and opportunities for improvement from a top-down approach, focusing on occupation first (e.g., self-care activities, functional mobility, instrumental activities of daily living) and then drilling down to client factors and performance skills that are familiar in medical settings (e.g., assessment of range of motion, manual muscle testing, vision, and cognition).

Adult physical rehabilitation is the largest practice area in OT, as well as the one most closely aligned with the traditional medical model, resulting in constraints that can sometimes create tension and an unnecessary narrowing of OT's scope of practice. We have therefore chosen 13 studies that demonstrate the breadth and depth of OT practice provided to people within major diagnostic groups, across a variety of physical medicine and rehabilitation settings, and with an appreciation of how policy and regulatory issues can both support and confine clinical practice. To illustrate the full scope of OT in this practice area, we selected six studies that explore the distinct value and nature of occupation-based practice, four studies that highlight the critical need for participation in multiple contexts, and three studies that demonstrate the power of OT from a regulatory and policy perspective.

The studies that explore occupation-based practice start with the seminal work of Mattingly and Fleming, describing the unique features and aspects of clinical reasoning in OT. Other studies highlight the importance of occupation and activity-based interventions in various diagnostic areas: spinal cord injury (Ghaisas et al.), multiple sclerosis (Mathiowetz et al.), stroke (Trombly & Ma), cancer (Hunter et al.), and traumatic brain injury (Powell et al.).

Research highlighting the critical nature of participation in a variety of contexts includes an assessment of driving readiness (Dickerson), a qualitative study critically examining participation and performance from the disability communities' perspective (Hammel et al.), an exploratory randomized controlled trial combining cognitive retraining strategies and task-specific training to improve participation for individuals post-stroke (McEwen et al.), and the landmark paper by Law et al. establishing the Canadian Occupational Performance Measure as a foundational assessment for setting goals and measuring progress toward participation in everyday occupations.

We chose three studies that demonstrate the power of OT in regulatory and policy contexts given that OT services are generally subject to regulatory controls and are highly influenced by local, state, and national policy. One study analyzed the association of length of stay, recovery rate, and therapy minutes for patients recovering from hip fracture surgery, providing needed insight into factors impacting outcomes as rehabilitation shifts from volume to value-based care (Cogan et al.). Another demonstrated the benefit of early occupational and physical therapy for critically ill patients (Schweickert et al.). Lastly, Rogers et al. concluded that higher hospital spending on OT was the only spending category associated with lower readmission rates. At a time when hospital spending is challenged and budget priorities abound, evidence supporting policy decisions regarding OT in all contexts is needed and can be directly applied.

OT practice in physical disabilities and rehabilitation covers a broad range of populations, conditions, and settings. The studies chosen reflect that diversity but are not entirely representative of the full scope of OT practice in rehabilitation. Furthermore, these studies reveal that rehabilitation research is still primarily conducted among majority populations. Most participants in these studies were adults, especially older adults 45 years of age and above, and White. Four exceptions are noted, which included greater representation of Black and Hispanic individuals (Ghaisas et al. McEwen et al., Schweickert et al., Hammel et al.).

These 13 studies provide directly applicable insight into OT practice in physical rehabilitation settings. It is critical that OT practitioners foreground occupation in practice and clearly document the therapeutic benefits of its use.

Throughout this section, we hope to inspire OT practitioners and encourage them to continue to learn, grow, and further develop their practice to be powerful, occupation-based, centered on the client's participation, and recognized as distinctly valuable.

Reference

Gray, J. M. (1998). Putting occupation into practice: Occupation as ends, occupation as means. *Journal of Occupational Therapy, 52*(5), 354–364.

38

Lifestyle Changes and Pressure Ulcer Prevention in Adults with Spinal Cord Injury

JESUS DIAZ

This secondary analysis provided a first glimpse into issues that may contribute to positive and negative outcomes of a lifestyle intervention to prevent pressure ulcers. Through analysis of the case studies, we became aware of the complexity of participants' lives, the impact of the environment and events outside participants' control, and the role of the health care system in shaping participants' lifestyle and behaviors in response to pressure ulcers.

GHAISAS, S., PYATAK, E. A., BLANCHE, E., BLANCHARD, J., & CLARK, F.; PUPS II STUDY GROUP. (2015). Lifestyle changes and pressure ulcer prevention in adults with spinal cord injury in the Pressure Ulcer Prevention Study lifestyle intervention. *American Journal of Occupational Therapy, 69,* Article 6901290020.

Original Paper: http://dx.doi.org/10.5014/ajot.2015.012021

Research Question: How do lifestyle choices contribute to the risk of developing pressure ulcers?

Funding: The National Institutes of Health, the Eunice Kennedy Shriver National Institute of Child Health and Human Development, and the National Center for Medical Rehabilitation Research

Year Study Began: 2012

Year Study Published: 2015

Study Location: Downey, CA

Who Was Studied: This study analyzed data from 25 participants in the intervention arm of the Pressure Ulcer Prevention Study II (PUPS II) randomized controlled trial who developed pressure ulcers during the intervention. Study participants were English- or Spanish-speaking adults with spinal cord injury and a history of serious pressure ulcers.

Who Was Excluded: The study reviewed all participants who completed the intervention for PUPS II ($n = 47$). Participants were excluded from the analysis if they did not develop pressure ulcers during the intervention ($n = 17$), had poor adherence (<17%) to the lifestyle intervention ($n = 2$), or had irregular patterns of lifestyle and behavior change that could not be categorized ($n = 3$).

How Many Participants: 25

Study Overview: This paper presents a secondary analysis examining the relationship between lifestyle change and pressure ulcer development among recipients of a pressure ulcer prevention intervention. Data analysis followed a four-step process (Figure 38.1). First, participants were classified based on the relationship between their lifestyle changes and pressure ulcer status. Second, data from several participants were organized into provisional case studies to explore the relationship between lifestyle changes and pressure ulcers. Third, to validate these patterns, treatment notes for all participants were reviewed and categorized into previously identified patterns. Finally, all cases were reviewed to confirm the categories assigned to participants, and exemplary cases were identified that best represented the four identified patterns between lifestyle changes and the formation of pressure ulcers.

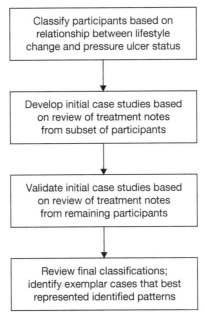

Figure 38.1. Overview of the study design.

Study Intervention: PUPS II was a 12-month lifestyle-focused intervention administered by occupational therapists through in-home visits and phone calls. The intervention was manualized and structured around six different modules with an emphasis on incorporating pressure ulcer prevention habits and routines into their daily lives.

Endpoints: Relationship between lifestyle and behavior changes and pressure ulcer status.

RESULTS

- There were four patterns identified through the analysis that characterized the relationship between lifestyle changes and pressure ulcer status:
  o *Positive lifestyle and behavior changes with positive changes in pressure ulcer status*: The majority of cases ($n = 19$) benefited from the intervention and demonstrated improvement of their pressure ulcer status without the need for surgical intervention.
  o *Positive lifestyle and behavioral changes with negative or no change in pressure ulcer status* ($n = 3$ cases)

- o *Minor or no lifestyle and behavior changes with positive changes in pressure ulcer status* ($n = 1$ case)
- o *Minor or no lifestyle and behavior change with negative or no change in pressure ulcer status* ($n = 2$ cases)
- Overall, when reviewing those who completed the intervention of PUPS II, 76% of participants did not develop pressure ulcers or saw improvements in their pressure ulcer status through lifestyle or behavior change informed by the intervention.
- The relationships between lifestyle and behavior changes are complex, and the patterns identified were not absolute.
- Due to the complexity of this relationship, additional factors such as medical complications, access to necessary equipment, environmental limitations, and unanticipated life circumstances need to be considered when addressing pressure ulcer development.

Criticisms and Limitations: This was a secondary analysis completed through an analysis of the interveners' treatment notes as interpreted by the authors. Since the treatment notes were not generated for this purpose and because of the limited number of cases reviewed, definitive conclusions cannot be made regarding whether the patterns were causative for pressure ulcer healing or lifestyle change.

Other Relevant Studies and Information:

- A subsequent paper discussed the results of the PUPS II randomized controlled trial and highlighted the challenges of preventing pressure ulcers in socioeconomically disadvantaged individuals (Carlson et al., 2019).
- Further analysis of participants who developed pressure ulcers during the PUPS II study indicated the importance of understanding a client's unique personal contexts while also providing them the skills to advocate for the services and equipment needed to improve care (Floríndez et al., 2020).
- A secondary analysis of participants in the PUPS II intervention trial who did not develop pressure ulcers revealed a range of protective factors, including potentially modifiable factors such as engagement in meaningful activities, self-advocacy skills, maintaining health-promoting behaviors, and accessing appropriate medical equipment (Sleight et al., 2019).

- A qualitative study of 20 adults with spinal cord injury identified eight lifestyle principles that were connected to pressure ulcer development: perpetual danger, change/disruption of routine, decay of prevention behaviors, lifestyle risk ratio, individualization, simultaneous presence of prevention awareness and motivation, lifestyle trade-offs, and access to needed care, services, and supports (Jackson et al., 2010).

Summary and Implications: Lifestyle factors and pressure ulcer development are interrelated and demonstrate a complex and dynamic relationship. As clinicians, it is important to consider the various factors, both modifiable and non-modifiable, that can potentially impact pressure ulcer development, such as medical complications, unexpected life circumstances, environmental components, and quality of the healthcare system, as well as community-based practices to comprehensively address lifestyle and environmental elements that increase risk.

CLINICAL CASE: ADDRESSING LIFESTYLE FACTORS FOR PRESSURE ULCER MANAGEMENT

Case History

Mario (he/him) is a 42-year-old Latino man who sustained a T1 spinal cord injury due to a gunshot wound and currently works as a concert promoter and community activist. He has a history of pressure ulcers on his right buttock that started after hospitalization following a car accident. Mario presents with challenges to performing pressure reliefs due to shoulder pain from the accident and having a body mass index of 32. He is currently dependent on others to perform skin checks and pressure reliefs and lacks appropriate medical equipment to decrease his risks for pressure ulcers. Mario is also dealing with depression after recently losing his son to gang violence. How would an occupational therapist address these factors to assist in the prevention of pressure ulcers?

Suggested Answer

It is important to work collaboratively with Mario to identify risks and establish goals to help reduce the risk of pressure ulcers. Lifestyle changes to help Mario improve his eating habits and increase physical activity can support weight loss to facilitate pressure reliefs. In order to address his shoulder pain, the occupational therapist can facilitate pain management strategies and help identify alternative methods for performing wheelchair mobility, skin checks, and pressure reliefs and incorporate them into his daily routines. Providing

Mario with opportunities to strengthen self-advocacy skills can support improved access to medical equipment. It is important to ensure that Mario is able to appropriately use and maintain his medical equipment in the home. Finally, it will also be crucial to support Mario's management of his depression through exploration and engagement in meaningful occupations and roles and by connecting him with the necessary community supports.

References

Carlson, M., Vigen, C. L., Rubayi, S., Blanche, E. I., Blanchard, J., Atkins, M., Bates-Jensen, B., Garber, S. L., Pyatak, E. A., Diaz, J., Floríndez, L. I., Hay, J. W., Mallinson, T., Unger, J. B., Azen, S. P., Scott, M., Cogan, A., & Clark, F. (2019). Lifestyle intervention for adults with spinal cord injury: Results of the USC–RLANRC Pressure Ulcer Prevention Study. *The Journal of Spinal Cord Medicine, 42*(1), 2–19.

Floríndez, L. I., Carlson, M. E., Pyatak, E., Blanchard, J., Cogan, A. M., Sleight, A. G., Hill, V., Diaz, J., Blanche, E., Garber, S. L., & Clark, F. A. (2020). A qualitative analysis of pressure injury development among medically underserved adults with spinal cord injury. *Disability and Rehabilitation, 42*(15), 2093–2099.

Jackson, J., Carlson, M., Rubayi, S., Scott, M. D., Atkins, M. S., Blanche, E. I., Saunders-Newton, C., Mielke, S., Wolfe, M. K., & Clark, F. A. (2010). Qualitative study of principles pertaining to lifestyle and pressure ulcer risk in adults with spinal cord injury. *Disability and Rehabilitation, 32*, 567–578. http://dx.doi.org/10.3109/0963828090 3183829

Sleight, A. G., Cogan, A. M., Hill, V. A., Pyatak, E. A., Díaz, J., Floríndez, L. I., Blanchard, J., Vigen, C., Garber, S. L., & Clark, F. A. (2019). Factors protecting against pressure injuries in medically underserved adults with spinal cord injury: A qualitative study. *Topics in Spinal Cord Injury Rehabilitation, 25*(1), 31–40. https://doi.org/10.1310/ sci2501-31

39

Energy Conservation Interventions for Multiple Sclerosis

REBECCA CUNNINGHAM

This randomized controlled trial supports the efficacy and effectiveness of [an energy conservation (EC) course] to decrease fatigue impact, and to increase self-efficacy and some aspects of quality of life. Thus, this EC course taught by occupational therapists is a legitimate non-pharmacological approach for managing fatigue for persons with [multiple sclerosis].

MATHIOWETZ, V. G., FINLAYSON, M. L., MATUSKA, K. M., CHEN, H. Y., & LUO, P. (2005). Randomized controlled trial of an energy conservation course for persons with multiple sclerosis. *Multiple Sclerosis, 11,* 592–601.

Research Question: What is the short-term efficacy and effectiveness of a 6-week energy conservation (EC) course on fatigue, self-efficacy, and quality of life in individuals living with multiple sclerosis (MS)?

Funding: The National Multiple Sclerosis Society

Year Study Began: 2002–2003

Year Study Published: 2005

Study Location: Illinois and Minnesota

Who Was Studied: Adults 18 years of age or older with a diagnosis of MS who self-identified as having moderate to severe fatigue (Fatigue Severity score of 4 or greater), were independently living in the community, were motivated to participate in the 6-week EC course, and displayed no more than mild cognitive impairment.

Who Was Excluded: Individuals were excluded if they were not able to read course materials in English and/or failed more than one subtest of the Neuropsychological Screening Battery for Multiple Sclerosis.

How Many Patients: 169

Study Overview: See Figure 39.1.

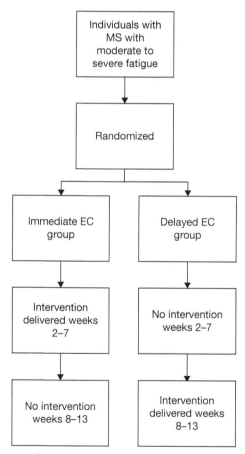

Figure 39.1. Overview of the study design.

Study Intervention: The 6-week EC course was delivered by trained occupational therapists in community settings. Twenty EC groups were completed, with each group consisting of 7–10 participants. Sessions were delivered once per week with a total of six sessions possible for attendance. Sessions were 2 hours in duration and consisted of lecture, discussion, short-term and long-term goal-setting, activity application, and home-based activities to support carryover into daily life. The course addressed the following conceptual areas: rest routines, communication, body mechanics, ergonomics, activity analysis and modifications, lifestyle balance, shifting expectations, and priority-setting. Participants who missed a session were given access to a self-learning module with application activities to support learning of the content. Per the crossover design, the immediate EC group participated during Weeks 2–7, and the delayed EC group participated during Weeks 8–13.

Follow-Up: Participants completed outcome measures at Weeks 1, 7, and 13.

Endpoints: Primary outcome measures were the Fatigue Impact Scale (FIS) and the Short Form-36 Health Survey (SF-36). The FIS measures the impact of fatigue on participants' lives, and the SF-36 measures participants' perceived health-related quality of life. The secondary outcome measure was the Self-Efficacy for Performing Energy Conservation Strategies Assessment. This outcome was designed for the study to measure participants' self-efficacy in their ability to perform 14 EC behaviors. The researchers completed between-groups intention-to-treat (ITT) analyses using two different approaches: last-observation-carried-forward (LOCF) and maximum likelihood methods, as well as compliers-only analyses on participants who completed at least five of six EC course sessions.

RESULTS

- When FIS and SF-36 outcomes were combined, the immediate EC group showed significant improvement in fatigue and quality of life across all analyses (Table 39.1).
- When the FIS and SF-36 were considered separately, significant differences were demonstrated for both outcomes in favor of the immediate EC group across all analyses.
- When each subscale of the FIS was considered individually, all were significant except the Cognitive subscale in the ITT LOCF and compliers-only analyses, in favor of the immediate EC group.
- When each subscale of the SF-36 was considered individually, the immediate EC group showed significant improvement in Vitality (all

analyses), Role-Physical (both ITT analyses), and Mental Health scores
(ITT likelihood).

- Participants reported average implementation of 9.2 new EC strategies due
  to participation in the EC course. The self-efficacy score was significantly
  higher from pre-intervention to post-intervention across all analyses.
- The attrition rate was 23% or $n = 39$, which was higher than anticipated by
  the researchers when compared to similar studies.
- Based on participant comments, the authors concluded that peer support
  within the group format provided opportunities for problem-solving,
  reinforcement of successes, and encouragement, which supported
  participant self-efficacy with performance of EC strategies.

Table 39.1. SUMMARY OF STUDY KEY FINDINGS

Outcome	ITT Likelihood p Value	ITT LCOF p Value	Compliers Only p Value
3FIS subscales + SF-36 subscales	<0.000*	0.001*	0.004*
3FIS subscales	0.001*	0.006*	0.003*
FIS: Cognitive	0.009*	0.017	0.037
FIS: Physical	0.000*	0.000*	0.000*
FIS: Social	0.000*	0.001*	0.002*
8SF-36 subscales	<0.000*	0.000*	0.002*
SF-36: Physical Function	0.429	0.484	0.625
SF-36: Role-Physical	0.004*	0.005*	0.036
SF-36: Body Pain	0.410	0.707	0.936
SF-36: General Health	0.717	0.715	0.619
SF-36: Vitality	<0.000*	<0.000*	<0.000*
SF-36: Social Function	0.051	0.067	0.045
SF-36: Role-Emotional	0.068	0.086	0.112
SF-36: Mental Health	0.006*	0.016	0.020
Self-Efficacy	<0.000*	<0.000*	<0.000*

NOTE: Results have been rounded to the thousandth place.
*Significant finding.

Criticisms and Limitations: The results of the study cannot be generalized to
individuals with MS who have moderate to severe cognitive impairment. The
23% attrition rate was higher than anticipated, which impacts the power of the
analyses and makes it more challenging to identify significant between-group
differences. Due to the nature of the intervention, blinding of participants and
interventionists was not possible, which increases the risk of bias.

Other Relevant Studies and Information:

- One-year follow-up of the reviewed study showed maintenance of benefits gained since post-intervention, as well as significant improvement in the Cognitive FIS subscale, which was not significant at post-intervention (Mathiowetz et al., 2007).
- A similar 8-week EC course was delivered for individuals with progressive forms of MS with significant improvements in all FIS scores, which were maintained at 8 weeks post-intervention (Vanage et al., 2003).
- A telehealth application of an EC course protocol via conference calls for individuals with MS demonstrated significant improvements in fatigue impact but not fatigue severity, and in pooled samples showed benefit for fatigue impact, fatigue severity, and quality of life (Finlayson et al., 2011).
- One-to-one application of an EC protocol with individuals who have chronic conditions, including MS, demonstrated significant improvements in fatigue, self-efficacy and quality of life, which were maintained at 6 weeks post-intervention (Van Heest et al., 2017).

Summary and Implications: This randomized controlled trial supports the efficacy and effectiveness of a 6-week EC course delivered by occupational therapists for improving fatigue impact, self-efficacy, and some areas of quality of life in individuals with MS who self-identify as having moderate to severe fatigue. Findings are generalizable to individuals with no more than mild cognitive impairment as those with moderate to severe cognitive impairment were excluded from the study. Due to short-term and potential long-term benefits, occupational therapists should consider recommending and delivering group fatigue management interventions to optimize care for their patients with MS.

CLINICAL CASE: OCCUPATIONAL THERAPY AND EC PROGRAMS FOR MS

Case History

Sasha (she/her), a 38-year-old woman arrives at an outpatient clinic to initiate occupational therapy services. During evaluation, the patient reports she has been living with MS for over 10 years, experiences moderate levels of fatigue that can fluctuate to severe, and recognizes that heat sensitivity and overexertion make symptoms worse. Sasha denies sleep deficits and comorbidities.

She reports that fatigue significantly impacts participation in meaningful occupations including work, exercise, and cooking. Additionally, the patient describes difficulty keeping plans with friends due to frequent cancellations related to her fatigue presentation, which is resulting in feelings of social isolation. She states, "I've basically stopped making plans with my friends because my fatigue feels unpredictable." Upon screening, the patient's cognition is within normal limits.

Suggested Answer

The current study and articles included in the relevant studies section of this chapter suggest that group EC intervention delivery benefits fatigue, self-efficacy, and quality of life in individuals living with fatigue secondary to MS. The patient in this case study is typical of one who experiences MS-related fatigue. Due to Sasha's cognitive abilities demonstrated during screening and self-identified moderate fatigue severity, it is appropriate to refer her to a group EC course. Depending on the needs and proximity to courses, the occupational therapist (OT) should review both in-person and virtual options with the patient. Additionally, it is encouraged that the OT plan on reinforcing skills learned in the EC course during their outpatient plan of care to support carry-over across occupations and contexts.

References

Finlayson, M., Preissner, K., Cho, C., & Plow, M. (2011). Randomized trial of teleconference-delivered fatigue management program for people with multiple sclerosis. *Multiple Sclerosis Journal*, 17(9), 1130–1140.

Mathiowetz, V. G., Matuska, K. M., Finlayson, M. L., Luo, P., & Chen, H. Y. (2007). One-year follow-up to a randomized controlled trial of an energy conservation course of persons with multiple sclerosis. *International Journal of Rehabilitation Research*, 30(4), 305–313.

Vanage, S. M., Gilbertson, K. K., & Mathiowetz, V. (2003). Effects of energy conservation course on fatigue impact for persons with progressive multiple sclerosis. *American Journal of Occupational Therapy*, 57:315–323.

Van Heest, K. N. L., Mogush, A. R., & Mathiowetz, V. G. (2017). Centennial topics: Effects of a one-to-one fatigue management course for people with chronic conditions and fatigue. *American Journal of Occupational Therapy*, 71, Article 7104100020.

40

Effects of Occupational Therapy for Persons with Stroke on Restoration of Roles, Tasks, and Activities and on Remediation of Impairments

A Systematic Review and Meta-Analysis

ALLISON CHU

We conclude that occupational therapy effectively improves participation and activity after stroke and recommend that therapists use structured instruction in specific, client-identified activities, appropriate adaptations to enable performance, practice within a familiar context, and feedback to improve client performance.

TROMBLY, C. A., & MA, H. I. (2002). A synthesis of the effects of occupational therapy for persons with stroke, part I: Restoration of roles, tasks, and activities. *American Journal of Occupational Therapy, 56*(3), 250–259.

MA, H. I., & TROMBLY, C. A. (2002). A synthesis of the effects of occupational therapy for persons with stroke, part II: Remediation of impairments. *American Journal of Occupational Therapy, 56*(3), 260–274.

Original Papers:

- Part I: https://doi.org/10.5014/ajot.56.3.250
- Part II: https://doi.org/10.5014/ajot.56.3.260

Research Question: What is the effectiveness of occupational therapy (OT) for persons who have had a stroke on the restoration of valued roles, tasks, and activities and the remediation of bodily impairment functions?

Funding: American Occupational Therapy Association

Year Study Began: Studies between 1980 and 2000

Year Study Published: 2002

Study Location: Boston University

Who Was Studied: This systematic review included only studies published in English, peer-reviewed journals between 1980 and 2000. Studies had to measure the effect of treatment on persons with stroke. Treatment had to be designated as OT, administered by an occupational therapist, or researched or reported by occupational therapists.

Who Was Excluded: The meta-analysis excluded studies that did not clearly provide distinct OT intervention or if the intervention providers were not occupational therapists. Studies were also excluded if the effects of intervention were not reported in functional terms or could not be attributed solely to OT.

How Many Studies: 36

Study Overview: This is a two-part synthesis of 36 studies examining the effects of OT to improve activity and participation and to reduce impairments for persons with stroke. The first part synthesized research findings for the restoration of role participation and activity performance, while the second part synthesized research findings regarding the effects of OT to remediate the psychosocial, cognitive-perceptual, and sensorimotor impairments. The level of evidence and statistics for each study were examined and evaluated. The review was organized by therapeutic goals: restoration of roles, tasks, and activities (Part I) and remediation of impaired bodily functions (Part II).

Endpoints: Outcome variables were classified into the International Classification of Functioning, Disability, and Health categories of participation (role), activity (instrumental activities of daily living [IADLs] and basic activities of daily living [BADLs]), as well as structural and functional integrity (mental and physical abilities and capacities).

RESULTS

Part I: Restoration of Roles, Tasks, or Activities

- Fifteen studies addressed restoration of roles, tasks, or activities. Of these, three were classified as randomized controlled trials (RCTs; Level I) with high internal validity. Of the remaining 12 studies, seven were designated as RCTs (Level I) with one or more threats to internal validity, two as multiple group comparisons without randomization to treatment (Level II), and three as one-group pretest–posttest designs (Level III).
- *Participation in Life Roles*: Three studies concluded that the effect of OT on the restoration of role performance appeared to depend on dosage and goal specificity. Intervention that was longer in duration and higher in frequency and had more structure positively impacted role performance and satisfaction.
- *Activity (IADL)*: Eight studies examined the effects of various intensities of in-home or community-based therapy focused on task-specific practice on IADL performance. Improvement was noted in 16% more cases after task-specific practice in a familiar context, especially in the home, compared to those conducted under the control conditions, either routine services or usual community OT care. No significant difference on IADL performance was found between task-specific practice and sensorimotor intervention; participants improved significantly after both interventions.
- *Activity (BADL)*: Five of the nine studies reported significant improvement in BADL performance. Task-specific practice of client-identified activities in the client's home resulted in better performance of dressing and other self-care activities than no treatment.

Part II: Remediation of Impairments

- Twenty-nine studies addressed remediation of impairments of bodily functions. Of these, eight were RCTs with high internal validity (Level I). Of the remaining 21 studies, nine were designated as RCTs (Level I) with one or more threats to internal validity, nine as multiple group comparisons without randomization to treatment (Level II), two as one-group pretest–posttest designs (Level III), and one as a single-case study (Level IV) replicated over several participants, allowing meta-analytic synthesis.
- *Psychosocial*: Four studies measured the effect of OT on depression and psychological well-being after stroke as a secondary outcome of interventions to improve BADL and IADL skills in the home. Effect sizes

were in the small to medium range, warranting more focused research in this area.

- *Cognitive-Perceptual*: Eight studies addressed cognitive-perceptual abilities and capacities, including learning ability. Homemaking tasks as therapy resulted in 36%–46% greater improvement rates than paper-and-pencil tasks or arts and crafts to improve some cognitive functions. Focused visual scanning training for clients with unilateral neglect was more effective than generalized intervention. Intervention involving forced awareness of increased space, task-specific practice, and use of consistent strategies to accomplish functional activities improved cognitive-perceptual abilities after stroke.

- *Sensorimotor*: Fifteen studies examined the effect of OT on motor capacities. An effect of meaningfulness of activity on endurance was noted by increased participation of clients during preferred versus non-preferred activities. Two studies concluded that exercises to recruit motor units in the prime mover were insufficient for regaining movement. However, practice of movement to achieve a specific goal had small to moderate positive effects on range of motion compared with control conditions. Tasks that used actual objects within a functional goal and contextual support enhanced the organization and coordination of movements of persons with or without stroke.

Criticisms and Limitations: It is difficult to differentiate OT's specific effect on restoration of role performance from that of other professions as restoration of role performance involves the whole rehabilitation team. Other concurrent factors influencing the effect of OT on participation in BADL and IADL during the acute stage poststroke include spontaneous recovery and co-interventions.

Other Relevant Studies and Information:

- An evidence-based review found that a variety of interventions are effective at improving aspects of occupational performance in stroke survivors who have residual motor impairments (Nilsen et al., 2015). The evidence suggested that repetitive task practice, constraint-induced or modified constraint-induced movement therapy, strengthening and exercise, mental practice, virtual reality, mirror therapy, and action observation can improve upper extremity function, balance, mobility, activity, and participation. Many of the studies reviewed involved training of the impaired arm and hand using goal-directed and individualized tasks as well as frequent repetitions of task-related or task-specific movements, further supporting the importance and effectiveness of task-oriented training (Stoykov & Corcos, 2009).

- An evidence-based review supported the use of occupation-based interventions to improve occupational performance, especially ADLs, after stroke (Wolf et al., 2015). More evidence supported the use of occupation-based interventions than impairment remediation approaches to improve ADL performance in the inpatient, outpatient, and community settings (Almhdawi et al., 2016; Song, 2015). There was limited to no evidence supporting occupation-based interventions to address other areas of occupation beyond ADLs and IADLs, such as leisure, social participation, and rest or sleep poststroke. The underemphasis within OT practice and research on IADL performance, leisure, social participation, rest and sleep, and work and productivity highlights the need for further research on these domains.

Summary and Implications: OT effectively improves BADL and IADL performance, role restoration, and bodily function impairment in persons who have had a stroke. According to the studies reviewed in this synthesis, key therapeutic mechanisms include the provision of opportunities for practice of client-preferred activities, contextual familiarity, structured and goal-specific teaching of activity skills and strategies, and provision of necessary adaptations and training in the use of the adaptations.

CLINICAL CASE: DETERMINING THE MOST EFFECTIVE OT TREATMENT APPROACH TO IMPROVE PARTICIPATION IN IADLS AFTER A STROKE

Case History

Martin (he/him) is a 78-year-old man who sustained a right cerebrovascular accident with resultant left hemiparesis. After a 2-week inpatient rehabilitation program at the hospital, he was discharged to his home with his wife as his primary caregiver. He is a retired civil engineer and enjoys playing golf, taking walks in his neighborhood, doing yard work, and using FaceTime to stay in touch with his adult children and grandchildren. Martin was referred to outpatient OT to continue with his recovery process and address his decreased participation in IADLs, specifically home management and driving, and decreased left upper extremity motor control. Which intervention approaches would be most effective for this client?

Suggested Answer

Involving Martin in the development of his OT program by encouraging him to identify and prioritize the BADLs and IADLs he would like to focus on will not only contribute to the restoration of his former roles but also guide the task-specific training approaches to be used in order to achieve optimal therapeutic gains. Identifying specific therapeutic activities, such as using technology and doing yard work, will provide opportunities for repetitive task practice in real-world contexts. Depending on the clinical presentation of Martin's left hemiparesis, a variety of possible intervention approaches should be considered including repetitive task practice, constraint-induced movement therapy, bilateral training, strengthening and exercise, virtual reality, mirror therapy, and neuromuscular electrical stimulation to improve his upper extremity function, balance, functional mobility, and overall participation in activities. Providing intensive motor training within the context of functional activities, variable practice, and intermittent feedback will enable Martin to achieve optimal functional performance.

References

Almhdawi, K. A., Mathiowetz, V. G., White, M., & delMas, R. C. (2016). Efficacy of occupational therapy task-oriented approach in upper extremity post-stroke rehabilitation. *Occupational Therapy International, 23*, 444–456. https://doi.org/10.1002/oti.1447

Ma, H. I., & Trombly, C. A. (2002). A synthesis of the effects of occupational therapy for persons with stroke, part II: Remediation of impairments. *American Journal of Occupational Therapy, 56*(3), 260–274.

Nilsen, D. M., Gillen, G., Geller, D., Hreha, K., Osei, E., & Saleem, G. (2015). Effectiveness of interventions to improve occupational performance of people with motor impairments after stroke: An evidence-based review. *American Journal of Occupational Therapy, 69*, Article 6901180030. http://dx.doi.org/10.5014/ajot.2015.011965

Song, G. B. (2015). The effects of task-oriented versus repetitive bilateral arm training on upper limb function and activities of daily living in stroke patients. *Journal of Physical Therapy Science, 27*(5), 1353–1355. https://doi.org/10.1589/jpts.27.1353

Stoykov, M. E., & Corcos, D. M. (2009). A review of bilateral training for upper extremity hemiparesis. *Occupational Therapy International, 16*(3–4), 190–203. https://doi.org/10.1002/oti.277

Trombly, C. A., & Ma, H. I. (2002). A synthesis of the effects of occupational therapy for persons with stroke, part I: Restoration of roles, tasks, and activities. *American Journal of Occupational Therapy, 56*(3), 250–259.

Wolf, T. J., Chuh, A., Floyd, T., McInnis, K., & Williams, E. (2015). Effectiveness of occupation-based interventions to improve areas of occupation and social participation after stroke: An evidence-based review. *American Journal of Occupational Therapy, 69*, Article 6901180060. http://dx.doi.org/10.5014/ajot.2015.012195

41

Occupational Therapy and Adult Cancer Rehabilitation

STACEY MORIKAWA AND YASAMAN AMANAT

Physical activity can help reduce CRF [cancer-related fatigue], improve the quality of sleep, increase physical function, and increase HRQOL [health-related quality of life] regardless of type or stage of cancer. (Part 1)

Moderate to strong evidence indicates that addressing the psychosocial components of cancer survivorship is beneficial for survivors regardless of age or type or stage of cancer and can improve anxiety, depression and quality of life. (Part 2)

HUNTER, E. G., GIBSON, R. W., ARBESMAN, M., & D'AMICO, M. (2017). Systematic review of occupational therapy and adult cancer rehabilitation: Part 1. Impact of physical activity and symptom management interventions. *American Journal of Occupational Therapy*, 71(2), 7102100030p1–7102100030p11.

HUNTER, E. G., GIBSON, R. W., ARBESMAN, M., & D'AMICO, M. (2017). Systematic review of occupational therapy and adult cancer rehabilitation: Part 2. Impact of multidisciplinary rehabilitation and psychosocial, sexuality, and return-to-work interventions. *American Journal of Occupational Therapy*, 71(2), 7102100040p1–7102100040p8.

Original Papers:

- Part 1: https://doi.org/10.5014/ajot.2017.023564
- Part 2: https://doi.org/10.5014/ajot.2017.023572

Research Question: What is the effectiveness of cancer rehabilitation interventions within the scope of occupational therapy practice to address the activity and participation needs of adult cancer survivors in activities of daily living, instrumental activities of daily living, work, leisure, social participation, and rest and sleep?

Funding: American Occupational Therapy Association (AOTA) Evidence-Based Practice Project

Year Study Began: Studies between 1995 and 2014

Year Study Published: 2017

Study Location: Systematic review of national data

Who Was Studied: The review included peer-reviewed scientific articles on adults with cancer and within the scope of practice of occupational therapy.

Who Was Excluded: The review excluded data from presentations, conference proceedings, non-peer-reviewed research literature, and dissertations and theses. It also excluded studies focusing on caregivers, family members, or friends rather than cancer survivors; studies of childhood cancer; and interventions that required an academic degree other than occupational therapy. Evidence determined to be at "Level IV and V" standard, which included descriptive studies, case reports, and expert opinion, was excluded from review.

How Many Studies: 138

Study Overview: The review authors, in collaboration with the methodology, consultant, AOTA staff, and the advisory group, developed the research question and search terms. The Cochrane risk-of-bias guidelines was used to assess the risk of bias of individual studies. The systematic review followed Preferred Reporting Items for Systematic Reviews and Meta-Analyses guidelines. In addition, risk of bias was assessed using the Assessment of Multiple Systematic Reviews system (Figure 41.1).

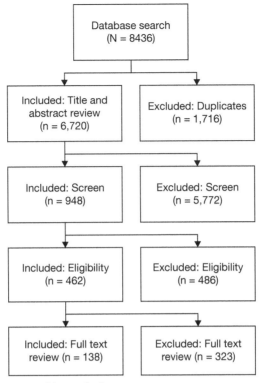

Figure 41.1. Overview of the study design.

Endpoints: Following synthesis of the articles, themes were identified as follows: interventions for physical activity, symptom management, psychosocial, multidisciplinary rehabilitation programs, sexuality, and return to work.

RESULTS

- Strong evidence was found that exercise is safe and beneficial for the majority of cancer types, at all stages, and regardless of age.
- Moderate evidence indicates that exercise improves health-related quality of life for some survivors.
- Strong evidence was found that exercise reduces cancer-related fatigue and increases quality of life.
- While the strength of the evidence is limited by the quality of the studies, there was moderate evidence to support the use of complementary and alternative medicine to improve quality of life and mental health outcomes.

- Strong evidence was found that multidisciplinary rehabilitation programs benefit survivors with many types of cancer before and after treatment. These programs resulted in improved function and participation regardless of type of cancer, stage of cancer, or age of individual.
- There is strong evidence indicating that psychosocial strategies, including cognitive-behavioral and educational interventions, decrease anxiety greater than 3 months following cancer treatment and depression 1–3 months following cancer treatment.
- There is limited evidence supporting the effectiveness of couple-based and psychoeducational interventions. There is limited research on interventions related to sexuality in patients with cancer.
- Moderate evidence showed that high-intensity exercise assisted in minimizing the decrease in work ability after cancer and treatment. However, further research in return to work for survivors is needed.

Criticisms and Limitations: Limitations of the systematic review included limitations in the individual studies' designs and methods. These included small sample sizes, short intervention periods, limited use of standardized assessments, and short follow-up periods. Additionally, few of the studies included occupation-based interventions or were specific in their outcomes regarding function and participation in meaningful daily activities.

Other Relevant Studies and Information:

- An article highlighting occupational therapy's role in cancer survivorship demonstrated the value of occupational therapy's unique perspective in treating the functional and psychosocial implications of cancer treatment on daily living and participation. It discussed occupational therapy's role in facilitating improved level of functioning and participation, including self-management, regardless of cancer survivors' stage of recovery (Baxter et al., 2017).
- An analysis evaluating the effects of exercise in patients with cancer found that exercise significantly improved quality of life and physical function. The results demonstrated that demographic, clinical, and intervention characteristics did not significantly moderate the effects found (Buffart et al., 2017).
- A cross-sectional descriptive study found that individuals had a significantly lower perceived quality of life during the first year of survivorship, including psychosocial complications such as depression

and anxiety. In addition, the results indicated moderate negative correlations between the reported functional deficits and quality of life. This study also highlighted occupational therapy's potential role in addressing these deficits (Hwang et al., 2015).

Summary and Implications: This analysis showed that physical activity is beneficial for people with cancer across all stages and regardless of age. The analysis also showed that occupational therapy intervention is useful in symptom management, including for pain, fatigue, and breathlessness. Furthermore, there is moderate to strong evidence supporting psychosocial interventions in combating anxiety and depression. Multidisciplinary rehabilitation programs were also shown to benefit survivors of varying oncological diagnoses.

CLINICAL CASE: IMPACTFUL OCCUPATIONAL THERAPY INTERVENTIONS IN ADULT CANCER REHABILITATION

Case History

Lucy (she/her), a 47-year-old woman with a diagnosis of breast cancer is seen for an occupational therapy evaluation in an outpatient clinic. The reasons for referral are listed as activities of daily living retraining, exercise program, and lymphedema. She is undergoing chemotherapy following a mastectomy and axillary lymph node dissection 7 months ago. During the evaluation, Lucy expresses concerns about the appropriateness of participating in physical activity, and she fears that this will exacerbate her lymphedema. She shares that this uncertainty has been causing her increased feelings of anxiousness, contributing to decreased participation in prior activities. As the treating occupational therapist, how would you respond?

Suggested Answer

The systematic review highlights the benefits of physical activity and importance of psychosocial intervention in adult cancer rehabilitation. Using the Hunter et al. analysis as a basis for discussion, the occupational therapist should discuss the benefits of exercise such as improved sleep and physical function and reduced cancer-related fatigue. In addition, the occupational therapist can assist in reducing the associated anxiety by reiterating that research suggests that exercise is not found to exacerbate lymphedema. Furthermore, psychosocial interventions, such as cognitive-behavioral and educational interventions, should be integrated into her care to reduce anxiety and increase quality of life, as highlighted in the systematic review. As analysis showed in the systematic review, the mentioned interventions are effective in facilitating increased engagement and participation in desired activities.

References

Baxter, M. F., Newman, R., Longpré, S. M., & Polo, K. M. (2017). Occupational therapy's role in cancer survivorship as a chronic condition. *American Journal of Occupational Therapy*, *71*(3), 7103090010P1–7103090010P7. https://doi.org/10.5014/ajot.2017.713001

Buffart, L. M., Kalter, J., Sweegers, M. G., Courneya, K. S., Newton, R. U., Aaronson, N. K., Jacobsen, P. B., May, A. M., Galvão, D. A., Chinapaw, M. J., Steindorf, K., Irwin, M. L., Stuiver, M. M., Hayes, S., Griffith, K. A., Lucia, A., Mesters, I., van Weert, E., Knoop, H., . . . Brug, J. (2017). Effects and moderators of exercise on quality of life and physical function in patients with cancer: An individual patient data meta-analysis of 34 RCTs. *Cancer Treatment Reviews*, *52*, 91–104. https://doi.org/10.1016/j.ctrv.2016.11.010

Hwang, E. J., Lokietz, N. C., Lozano, R. L., & Parke, M. A. (2015). Functional deficits and quality of life among cancer survivors: Implications for occupational therapy in cancer survivorship care. *American Journal of Occupational Therapy*, *69*, Article 6906290010. http://dx.doi.org/10.5014/ajot.2015.015974

42

Why Occupation Matters for Survivors of Traumatic Brain Injury (TBI)

SAMIA H. RAFEEDIE

Current research provides evidence for the use of various intervention approaches across a range of settings to improve occupational and social participation outcomes for people who have sustained a TBI. Additional research is needed to determine the nature and extent of the contribution of occupational therapy within those treatment approaches and the specific occupational intervention approaches most likely to be effective for each individual client.

POWELL, J. M., RICH, T. J, & WISE, E. K. (2016). Effectiveness of occupation- and activity-based interventions to improve everyday activities and social participation for people with traumatic brain injury: A systematic review. *American Journal of Occupational Therapy, 70,* 7003180040p1–7003180040p9.

Original Paper: https://doi.org/10.5014/ajot.2016.020909

Research Question: The systematic review addresses the research question, "What is the evidence for the effectiveness of occupation- and activity-based interventions to improve everyday activities and areas of occupation and social participation for people with traumatic brain injury?" (p. 2).

Funding: Funding was not disclosed; however, the study was conducted as part of the American Occupational Therapy Association (AOTA) Evidence-Based Practice (EBP) Project.

Year Study Began: Studies between 2008 and 2013

Year Study Published: 2016

Study Location: Systematic review of national data

Who Was Studied: Inclusion criteria included papers published between 2008 and 2013 in peer-reviewed scientific journals written in English; at least 50% of participants in the study sample were adults diagnosed with TBI, and interventions were within the scope of practice of occupational therapy.

Who Was Excluded: The systematic review excluded qualitative studies and reports from presentations, conference proceedings, non-peer-reviewed research literature, dissertations, and theses.

How Many Studies: 19

Study Overview:

- Using the evidence hierarchy described by Sackett et al. (1996), descriptive outcome studies and case series designs (Level IV evidence) and case reports, narrative literature reviews, and consensus statements (Level V evidence) were included only when Level I (systematic reviews, meta-analyses, randomized controlled trials [RCTs]), Level II (two-group nonrandomized studies), and Level III (one-group nonrandomized studies) evidence was not found (Figure 42.1).

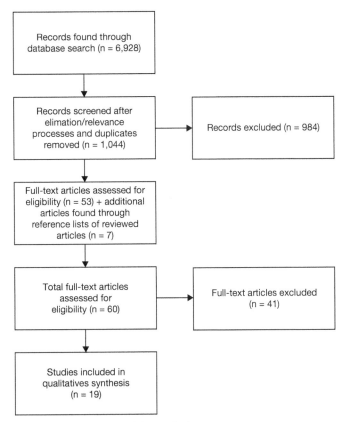

Figure 42.1. Overview of the study design.

- A methodology consultant to the AOTA EBP Project and AOTA staff
  identified the search terms in consultation with the review authors and
  the advisory group.

Follow-Up: Not applicable

Endpoints: Following synthesis of the articles, five categories of interventions
were identified: multidisciplinary and interdisciplinary intervention; community-
based rehabilitation; intervention using client-centered goals and relevant
contexts; social skills training and peer mentoring; and community mobility.

RESULTS

The qualitative synthesis resulted in five categories or themes describing types
of approaches or interventions that aim to improve performance of everyday

activities and areas of occupation and social participation for people who have sustained a TBI. Strong evidence indicates consistent results from well-conducted studies, typically at least two RCTs; moderate evidence was decided based on one RCT or two or more studies with lower levels of evidence; and limited evidence was used if there were few studies, flaws in the studies, or inconsistencies in the findings across separate studies.

Overall, moderate evidence supports a variety of interprofessional and community-based rehabilitation programs to improve occupational performance. Moderate evidence additionally indicates that activity-based, client-centered, and context-relevant strategies can improve occupational performance when delivered by an occupational therapist (OT).

1. Multidisciplinary and interdisciplinary treatment approaches

- Systematic review found moderate evidence that a variety of multidisciplinary and interdisciplinary approaches and programs are effective at improving performance and participation outcomes after a moderate to severe TBI, with strong evidence that there is not one single approach or setting that is more effective than another.
- Authors concluded that post-acute rehabilitation programs enhance community integration, especially for people with moderate to severe TBIs.
- Clients in more intensive programs appear to have better results than those in less structured, less intensive programs; such programs do not appear to be effective for those with mild TBI.

2. Community-based rehabilitation programs

- Five studies showed moderate evidence for the effectiveness of community-based rehabilitation programs of various types, with more intensive programs yielding better results, especially for those with moderate to severe TBIs.
- Comprehensive community-based rehabilitation programs may enhance daily life functioning and community reintegration, with the greatest support for holistic day treatment programs.
- Group intervention may demonstrate greater effects than individual therapy.
- Clients starting a community-based rehabilitation program within 1 year of injury showed the greatest improvements.
- Program costs were offset by savings in support costs within 2 years of starting a community-based rehabilitation program.

3. Treatment approaches using client-centered goals and relevant contexts
- There was moderate evidence that occupation- or activity-based interventions (individual and group) focused on client-centered goals and delivered in a client-relevant environmental context (regardless of setting) by an OT can improve occupational performance after TBI.

4. Social skills training and peer mentoring interventions
- There was limited evidence in support of social skills training programs and peer mentoring interventions improving some aspects of social skill functions, but they did not improve social participation globally.

5. Community mobility interventions
- There was limited evidence as to which treatment approaches should be used to improve community mobility for people who sustained a TBI.

Criticisms and Limitations: The review was limited by the small number of studies in total, the relatively high risk of bias, and low-quality designs of many studies. There was also a small or heterogeneous sample in many studies and limited reporting of intervention details in the studies reviewed. Therefore, conclusions are subject to bias, and interpretation should be done with caution.

Other Relevant Studies and Information:

- According to Williams et al. (2021), interdisciplinary teams enhance recovery outcomes for those with acquired brain injury and are increasingly goal-oriented toward independence, requiring patients to become involved with goal-setting and intervention processes.
- Engagement in rehabilitation therapies, like occupational therapy, is critical for successful outcomes; however, cognitive deficits must be addressed to maximize the effectiveness of individual interventions (Williams et al., 2021).
- Patients with higher levels of engagement will have greater gains than those who have lower engagement in rehabilitation therapy, who also experience increased health costs and long-term disability (Barello et al., 2012).
- Occupations such as activities of daily living (ADLs) and instrumental ADLs, as well as active social supports, contribute toward achieving satisfactory quality of life following TBI (Camp et al., 2020).
- Intervention provided by a coordinated team is more effective than uncoordinated intervention (Camp et al., 2020).

Summary and Implications: This systematic review found that OTs working in multidisciplinary and interdisciplinary teams using various intervention approaches across a range of settings would improve occupational and social participation outcomes for people recovering from TBI. Practitioners need to rely on clinical reasoning and expertise for best practice with decision-making, considering client preferences, program availability, and resource utilization. Additional research is needed to examine the specific effects of different occupational therapy approaches and interventions; optimal timing, frequency, and duration of intervention; as well as differential effects of client and injury characteristics on responsiveness to intervention.

CLINICAL CASE: OCCUPATIONAL THERAPY SERVICES FOLLOWING TBI—OCCUPATION MATTERS

Case History

Dennis (he/him) was admitted to the hospital emergency department with a severe TBI. He was involved in a drug deal altercation and survived several blows to the head. Upon admission, Dennis required total assistance for all ADLs and was dependent for all ADL transfers and mobility. He required supervision and assistance around the clock due to severe hemiplegia on the left side, visual impairments in the right eye, and significant cognitive dysfunction for foundational and higher-level cognitive skills. A percutaneous endoscopic gastronomy (PEG) tube was placed for nutrition, and he presented at a Rancho cognitive functioning Level IV (confused and agitated). Prior to admission, he lived in his car and was experiencing homelessness. The multidisciplinary rehabilitation team at the acute care hospital recommended inpatient acute rehabilitation. What kind of occupational therapy approaches and interventions will be prescribed?

Suggested Answer

At the inpatient acute rehabilitation unit, Dennis received comprehensive and intense interdisciplinary rehabilitation services from medicine, occupational therapy, physical therapy, speech and language pathology, nursing, dietary management, case management, recreational therapy, music therapy, and chaplain services 5 days a week for 3 hours per day. His OT supported him in achieving a daily routine of self-care activities requiring only minimal assistance before discharge. Dennis worked on self-care goals, including eating safely after the PEG tube was removed, learning how to transfer in and out of the bathtub, wheelchair dancing to his favorite music by Al Green, and engaging in occupation-based intervention that was client-centered and goal-directed. He received care for 4 weeks before being discharged to a community-based day program that provided intensive outpatient occupational therapy services, where he worked on instrumental ADLs and prepared to move into a group home with the help of his case manager.

References

Barello, S., Graffigna, G., & Vegni, E. (2012). Patient engagement as an emerging challenge for healthcare services: Mapping the literature. *Nursing Research and Practice, 2012,* Article 905934. https://doi.org/10.1155/2012/905934

Camp, A. L., Casteleijn, D., & Thupae, D. (2020). Responsiveness of the activity participation outcome measure in adult patients with traumatic brain injury in an acute private neurological rehabilitation setting in South Africa. *South African Journal of Occupational Therapy, 50*(2), 70–76. http://dx.doi.org/10.17159/2310-3833/2020/vol50no2a9

Powell, J. M., Rich, T. J., & Wise, E. K. (2016). Effectiveness of occupation- and activity-based interventions to improve everyday activities and social participation for people with traumatic brain injury: A systematic review. *American Journal of Occupational Therapy, 70,* 7003180040. http://dx.doi.org/10.5014/ajot.2016.020909

Sackett, D. L., Rosenberg, W. M. C., Muir Gray, J. A., Haynes, R. B., & Richardson, W. S. (1996). Evidence based medicine: What it is and what it isn't. *British Medical Journal, 312,* 71–72. http://dx.doi.org/10.1136/bmj.312.7023.71

Williams, M. W., Rapport, L. J., Hanks, R. A., & Parker, H. A. (2021). Engagement in rehabilitation therapy and functional outcomes among individuals with acquired brain injuries. *Disability and Rehabilitation, 43*(1), 33–41.

43

Clinical Reasoning among Occupational Therapists

JULIE MCLAUGHLIN GRAY

Clinical Reasoning Study

> Clinical reasoning for occupational therapists was **not** simply scientific reasoning, matching condition to therapy of choice; it went beyond that to a complex, practical reasoning aimed at determining "the good" for each particular client.
>
> MATTINGLY, C., & FLEMING, M. H. (1994). *Clinical reasoning: Forms of inquiry in a therapeutic practice.* F. A. Davis Company.

Original Work: https://www.fadavis.com/product/clinical-reasoning-forms-of-inquiry-in-a-therapeutic-practice

Research Question: How do occupational therapists (OTs) clinically reason in the midst of practice?

Funding: The American Occupational Therapy Association and the American Occupational Therapy Foundation

Year Study Began: 1986

Year Study Published: 1994

Study Location: Boston, MA

Who Was Studied: Fourteen OTs, seven of whom were senior therapists, from a variety of practice specializations, including acute neurology, cardiology, spinal cord injury, oncology, psychiatry, outpatient hand rehabilitation, and outpatient pediatrics.

Who Was Excluded: Practitioners in the setting who were not OTs.

How Many Participants: 154

Study Overview: The Clinical Reasoning Study took place from 1986 to 1990 and reflected a collaborative multidisciplinary effort including OTs and social scientists.

The researchers combined ethnographic methods with action research in order to study the clinical reasoning and experiences of OTs. Data generation involved observation and interviews of 14 occupational therapy (OT) practitioners in a variety of practice settings, including pediatrics, hand therapy, spinal cord injury, general physical disabilities, neurology, and psychiatry, within a large acute-care hospital that also included rehabilitation units. In addition to the primary researchers, seven faculty members from three different OT schools contributed to data analysis. The study encompassed three stages, as shown in Figure 43.1.

The shift from pure ethnography to action research occurred in stage three, during which the participating therapists were involved in structured analysis of video recordings of their clinical sessions.

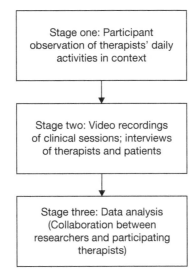

Figure 43.1. Overview of the study design.

Study Intervention: Not applicable

Follow-Up: Not applicable

Endpoints: Identification of themes related to how OTs conduct clinical reasoning.

RESULTS

- A primary outcome of this study was the discovery and description of various forms of clinical reasoning and signature aspects of OT practice, particularly those that are phenomenological in nature and not well described in biomedical theories and constructs. Secondarily, the authors revealed the "underground practice" of OTs—valuable work they did with patients but did not report or document—and the professional dilemmas experienced by many OTs while attempting to treat patients holistically within a medical context.
- Clinical reasoning in OT involves a practical form of reasoning that combines general theoretical principles along with consideration of the particular circumstances of the client and contextual factors.

- While OTs must consider and address the biological world of illness and disability, their primary concern is the illness experience or the "meaning of the disability for the person in his or her life" (p. 12).
- OTs experience tension between two conflicting paradigms in their clinical reasoning process: a mechanistic paradigm grounded in the concepts and theories of biomedicine and a phenomenological paradigm focused on values and lived experiences of their clients, representing their foremost professional commitment.
- In practice, OTs combine various forms of clinical reasoning in a seemingly fluid and concurrent manner, described by the authors as the "three-track mind":
  o *Procedural reasoning,* aimed at addressing functional limitations related to illness or disability
  o *Interactive reasoning,* focused on the collaborative relationship with the client(s)
  o *Conditional reasoning,* addressing the client's entire lifeworld and focused on creating meaningful experiences to impact or transform the client's sense of self in a positive way
- The work of OTs to address the phenomenological aspects of illness and disability, or specifically the client's lived experience of the condition, possesses narrative qualities in which therapists construct a "prospective treatment story," or stories of a desirable future that guide therapeutic approaches, sequences, and interpretation and represent a shared vision of the future between client and therapist, based upon the client's condition and life history.
- Many OTs experienced dilemmas in their practice related to tensions between core values of OT aimed at treating the whole person and the policies and norms of medical institutions, resulting in an "underground practice" of therapeutic activities and encounters they were less inclined to report or document. Such activities and encounters were typically perceived either as too unconventional in a biomedical context; as not billable, primarily when they did not specifically address the physical body; or as too difficult to describe in precise and measurable terms.

Criticisms and Limitations: Findings in the study reflect the experiences of OTs in a large teaching hospital and therefore may not reflect clinical reasoning experiences of OT practitioners who are certified OT assistants and/or who work in other practice settings, especially those that are less influenced by the medical model. While the Clinical Reasoning Study reflects seminal work in the profession, the findings should also be considered carefully in the present context, given the changing nature of the institutional systems and settings of care which have become more client-centered over time and the profession's evolving identity toward embracing, articulating, and studying the distinct value of occupation-centered care, both of which were intricately tied to the researchers' findings.

Other Relevant Studies and Information:

- Fleming (1991) wrote an article, further elaborating on findings from the Clinical Reasoning Study, that specifically contrasted the similarities and differences in the clinical reasoning in OT and in medicine. While hypothetical reasoning grounded in the scientific method is common to both professions, OTs integrated other forms of reasoning when their focus extended beyond the patient's medical problems to the personal, psychological, and social consequences of the condition.
- Several similar research projects have examined clinical reasoning in OT. Some of the most noteworthy and relevant include qualitative studies with similar approaches, albeit less extensive, that examined clinical reasoning among practitioners at different levels of education and in different settings:
  o Barris (1987) described a qualitative study that examined the clinical reasoning process of 19 OTs conducting initial evaluations in mental health settings.
  o Lyons and Crepeau (2001) used qualitative methods of interview and observation to study the clinical reasoning of an OT assistant with 16 years of experience. The researchers discovered evidence of the use of various types of reasoning by the OT assistant, including "pragmatic, procedural, interactive, conditional and narrative reasoning" (p. 577).
  o Munroe (1996) described findings from a qualitative study of the clinical reasoning of 30 OTs in Scotland who worked out of social work departments. Patterns of clinical reasoning identified consisted of reflection, decision-making, and reasoning.
  o Strong et al (1995) compared clinical reasoning between expert clinicians and fourth-year occupational therapy students and noted that experienced clinicians had more confidence, considered a broader range of factors, and were more scientific in their clinical reasoning.

- Several relevant articles written by contributors to the Clinical Reasoning Study were compiled in a special edition of the *American Journal of Occupational Therapy* in November 1991.
- A brief synopsis of the Clinical Reasoning Study design and essential findings can be found in Gilette and Mattingly (1987).

Summary and Implications: The Clinical Reasoning Study was a multiyear, in-depth examination of the clinical reasoning of OTs. Researchers observed, interviewed, and videotaped therapists from a variety of practice settings in a large teaching hospital and analyzed data collaboratively with the researchers and participating therapists. OTs fluidly combined procedural, interactive, and conditional reasoning in order to address patient needs within a biomedical context, with particular attention to the lived experience of illness and disability. This professional focus and commitment, contrary to biomedical norms, caused therapists to experience common dilemmas, sometimes resulting in an "underground practice" not apparent in their formal reports and documentation.

CLINICAL CASE: CHARLES AND THE CARBURETOR

Case History

Charles (he/him) was referred to hospital-based outpatient OT following a cerebrovascular accident (CVA). The OT evaluation, including an occupational history interview, revealed that Charles lived with his wife and was independent and active prior to his CVA. He was retired and very engaged in his leisure occupation of repairing and restoring antique cars. Since the stroke, Charles expressed minimal engagement in daily activities and routines. He relied on his wife for assistance with self-care and instrumental activities of daily living due to balance and mobility impairments and left hemiparesis with decreased coordination and function. The OT was concerned about Charles's lack of motivation and limited engagement in daily occupations. Charles did not want to discuss self-care goals and was focused on restoring upper extremity strength and function.

Suggested Answer

The OT decided not to focus on self-care goals, typically addressed in the rehabilitation context, and instead integrated Charles's passion for antique cars into his therapy. The OT designed sessions addressing Charles's goals of improving his balance and left upper extremity but through the activity of disassembling a carburetor, which was available in the OT department as a therapeutic tool. Charles was very engaged in the sessions and enthusiastically taught the OT about car mechanics while working. After a few visits, Charles communicated that he had resumed self-care and was engaged in other activities at home. The therapist's decisions demonstrated an artful integration of procedural, interactive, and clinical reasoning to impact Charles's physical function (mechanistic paradigm) and, most importantly, his lived experience and future vision as a person recovering from stroke (phenomenological paradigm).

References

Barris, R. (1987). Clinical reasoning in psychosocial occupational therapy: The evaluation process. *Occupational Therapy Journal of Research, 7*(3), 147–162.

Fleming, M. (1991). Clinical reasoning in medicine compared with clinical reasoning in occupational therapy. *American Journal of Occupational Therapy, 45*(11), 988–996. https://doi.org/10.5014/ajot.45.11.988

Gilette, N. P., & Mattingly, C. (1987). Clinical reasoning in occupational therapy. *American Journal of Occupational Therapy, 41*(6), 399–400.

Lyons, K. D., & Crepeau, E. B. (2001). The clinical reasoning of an occupational therapy assistant. *American Journal of Occupational Therapy, 55*(5), 577–581. https://doi.org/ 10.5014/ajot.55.5.577

Munroe, H. (1996). Clinical reasoning in community occupational therapy. *The British Journal of Occupational Therapy, 59*(5), 196–202. https://doi.org/10.1177/0308022 69605900502

Strong, J., Gilbert, J., Cassidy, S., & Bennett, S. (1995). Expert clinicians' and students' views on clinical reasoning in occupational therapy. *The British Journal of Occupational Therapy, 58*(3), 119–123. https://doi.org/10.1177/030802269505800309

44

Can the Assessment of Motor and Process Skills Predict Behind-the-Wheel Driving Performance?

ANA VERRAN

Because driving is an instrumental activity of daily living within the domain of occupational therapy practice, practitioners should be able to accurately determine who is a safe driver, who is at risk for unsafe driving, and who needs further evaluation by a specialist. The results of this pilot study strongly support this position.

DICKERSON, A. E., REISTETTER, T., DAVIS, E. S., & MONAHAN, M. (2011). Evaluating driving as a valued instrumental activity of daily living. *American Journal of Occupational Therapy*, 65(1), 64–75.

Original Paper: https://doi.org/10.5014/ajot.2011.09052

Research Question: Does an occupational therapy instrumental activity of daily living (IADL) assessment accurately identify individuals who pass, fail, or need restrictions, as indicated by a driver rehabilitation specialist (DRS)–administered behind-the-wheel (BTW) assessment?

Funding: East Carolina University

Year Study Began: 2006

Year Study Published: 2011

Study Location: East Coast of United States

Who Was Studied: Participants were predominantly White (81%) and female (56%), with a mean age of 70.22 ± 14.35 years. Thirteen were considered healthy community-living older adults, and the remaining 42 participants had diagnoses including cerebrovascular accident, traumatic brain injury, cognitive impairments or dementia, cardiac problems, and arthritis.

Who Was Excluded: Non-English speakers, novice drivers, persons needing adaptive driving equipment, those unable to provide written informed consent, and those unable to complete BTW, clinical, and IADL assessments were excluded.

How Many Patients: 55

Study Overview: The study compared the association between the Assessment of Motor and Process Skills (AMPS), an in-clinic assessment, and the gold standard BTW assessments, to identify whether the AMPS adequately discriminated between individuals who could safely drive and those who required driving restrictions (Figure 44.1).

Convenience samples drawn from Center A/Center B

Data analysis to compare BTW driving performance with performance on AMPS motor and process scales

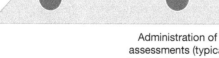

Administration of assessments (typical in-clinic tools used in driving evaluations, AMPS to assess IADL, and BTW)

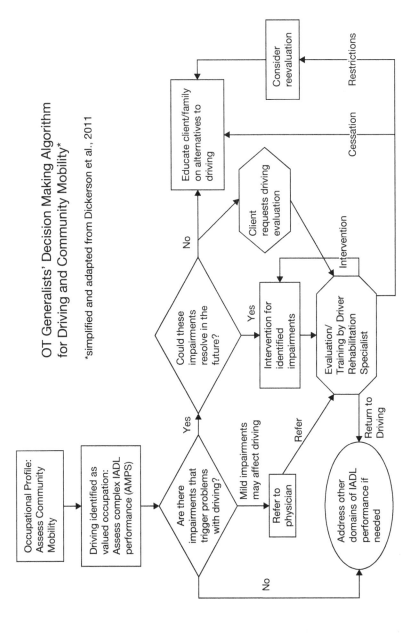

OT Generalists' Decision Making Algorithm for Driving and Community Mobility*

*simplified and adapted from Dickerson et al., 2011

Figure 44.1. Overview of the study design.

Endpoints:

Primary outcomes:

- IADL performance, as measured by the AMPS motor and process subscales
- Driving ability, as measured by a BTW assessment administered by a DRS

RESULTS

- Scores on the AMPS process scale were significantly associated with BTW assessment, with higher AMPS process scores associated with passing, lower with failure, and mid-range with restrictions on the BTW assessment.
- Process scores were significantly different between participants who passed and those who failed ($p < 0.01$) and between those with restrictions and those who failed ($p = 0.01$). There were no significant differences between participants who passed and those who received restrictions.
- AMPS motor scale scores were not associated with BTW assessments.
- The relationship between age and AMPS scores or BTW driving assessment was not significant; significant gender differences in AMPS process scores were demonstrated but were adjusted for in the analyses.
- Results suggest that AMPS process scores can accurately differentiate between individuals who pass or receive restrictions on a BTW assessment compared to those who fail a BTW assessment.
- These findings informed development of an algorithm for general practice occupational therapists that included IADL observations to guide decision-making about whether additional evaluation by a DRS was necessary to determine fitness to drive.

Criticisms and Limitations: The study included a relatively small number of participants from separate centers; results may not generalize to different populations. Administration of the BTW and AMPS assessments involved different driving evaluation specialists and calibrated AMPS testers. In addition,

BTW assessments were not completely standardized due to differences in community environments between the centers.

Other Relevant Studies and Information:

- DRSs have identified several barriers to developing an effective system for older driver evaluations. Barriers exist at the level of the individual (high time/cost investments for specialty training), relationships (inadequate collaborations with physicians/driver licensing agencies), community (uncertain sustainability of driving programs, need for alternative transportation resources), and society (low reimbursement levels, varying state requirements for reporting/liability, relationship between the Association for Driver Rehabilitation Specialists and the American Occupational Therapy Association) (Jones et al., 2016).
- Driving simulation and self-reported changes in driving proficiency were supported as methods of early identification of drivers meriting review (Vardaki et al., 2016).
- Individual tools measuring cognition, vision, perception, or physical ability individually are insufficient to determine fitness to drive. BTW assessment remains the evaluation gold standard, but there is emerging evidence for utilization of complex IADL observation and driving simulation as evaluation tools (Dickerson et al., 2014).
- Visual acuity, range of motion, strength, and fine motor coordination are assessed by most specialists; but there is no consistency in cognitive assessments used. BTW performance is primarily used for making a fitness to drive recommendation but lacks guidelines (Dickerson, 2013).

Summary and Implications: Results from this study suggest that occupational therapists can accurately determine who is a safe driver, who is at risk for unsafe driving, and who needs further evaluation by a DRS by utilizing a structured observation of other IADLs. Using IADL assessment to guide specialist referrals supports optimal utilization of scarce driver rehabilitation specialist resources. A decision-making algorithm was developed using the findings of this study to guide occupational therapists in determining whether to make a specialist referral.

CLINICAL CASE: USING IADL OBSERVATIONS TO DECIDE WHETHER TO REFER FOR SPECIALIZED DRIVING ASSESSMENT

Case History

Claire (she/her), an 87-year-old female with a medical history of chronic obstructive pulmonary disease, was in a stuporous state for 2 days following bowel resection surgery for a colon stricture. Two weeks after surgery she was discharged to a skilled nursing facility, where she remained for a week. She then transitioned to an assisted living facility for another 3 months before returning home with family assistance. Two months later, she began home health occupational and physical therapy to evaluate her ability to live independently and improve her limited endurance. During a home health session with her generalist occupational therapist, Claire expressed a desire to resume driving. Prior to her medical crisis, she drove to medical appointments, grocery and department stores, and her church and women's club activities.

Suggested Answer

The generalist occupational therapist used the AMPS to assess the quality of Claire's performance during a selected cooking task. Some difficulties with Claire's motor skills in sustaining performance and with her process skills in adapting her performance were observed. The generalist designed an intervention program to address these issues for home IADL performance but was unsure how the observed difficulties would impact Claire's ability to drive safely and independently. The clinical reasoning algorithm outlined in this article was used to determine that a referral to a DRS was indeed warranted. Following clinical and BTW assessments, the specialist occupational therapist recommended driver training to refresh Claire's knowledge of driving rules and regulations, followed by driving with restrictions (surface streets in immediate neighborhood, familiar routes, daylight hours, and off-peak traffic times).

References

Dickerson, A. E. (2013). Driving assessment tools used by driver rehabilitation specialists: Survey of use and implications for practice. *American Journal of Occupational Therapy*, 67(5), 564–573. https://doi.org/10.5014/ajot.2013.007823" https://doi.org/10.5014/ajot.2013.007823

Dickerson, A. E., Meuel, D. B., Ridenour, C. D., & Cooper, K. (2014). Assessment tools predicting fitness to drive in older adults: A systematic review. *American Journal of*

Occupational Therapy, 68(6), 670–680. https://doi.org/10.5014/ajot.2014.011833"
https://doi.org/10.5014/ajot.2014.011833

Jones, J., Dickerson, A., Flaten, H. K., Belmashkan, S., & Betz, M. E. (2016). Driving rehabilitation specialists' perspectives on older driver evaluations. *American Journal of Occupational Therapy, 70*(2), 7002270010p1–7002270010p7. https://doi.org/10.5014/ajot.2016.016915" https://doi.org/10.5014/ajot.2016.016915

Vardaki, S., Dickerson, A. E., Beratis, I., Yannis, G., & Papageorgiou, S. G. (2016). Simulator measures and identification of older drivers with mild cognitive impairment. *American Journal of Occupational Therapy, 70*(2), 7002270030p1–7002270030p10. https://doi.org/10.5014/ajot.2016.017673" https://doi.org/10.5014/ajot.2016.017673

45

Participation and Performance Are Not Synonymous

How Traditional Assessment Measures Fail the Disability Community

SAMIA H. RAFEEDIE

An Insider Perspective on Participation

The overwhelming message coming from the focus groups of people with disabilities was that no defined set of societal roles or social activities would be appropriate for all or indicative of "full" participation. Any effort to measure objective participation would have to be flexible enough to deal with the fact that different people will need, desire and endorse different aspects of participation and that very different patterns of participation can still reflect full participation.

HAMMEL, J., MAGASI, S., HEINEMANN, H., WHITENECK, G., BOGNER, J., & RODRIGUEZ, E. (2008). What does participation mean? An insider perspective from people with disabilities. *Disability and Rehabilitation, 30*(19), 1445–1460.

Original Paper: https://doi.org/10.1080/09638280701625534

Research Question: The purpose of this qualitative research study was to identify and describe indicators of participation from the perspective of individuals
with disabilities and to develop participation indicators that could be used to
guide assessment and program development. What are the qualitative indicators
of participation from the perspectives of individuals with disabilities and what
are the participation indicators that could be used to guide assessment and program development?

Funding: National Institute on Disability and Rehabilitation Research through
the Rehabilitation Research and Training Center on Measuring Rehabilitation
Outcomes and Effectiveness

Year Study Began: 2002

Year Study Published: 2008

Study Location: Illinois and Colorado

Who Was Studied: People with diverse types of disability, age, gender, race, and
ethnicity, who were either living in community-based settings or anticipating return to the community after rehabilitation or hospitalization.

Who Was Excluded: People living in institutional settings were not included.

How Many Patients: 63

Study Overview: Participants were asked five guiding questions that were developed in collaboration with community partners to frame the research:

1. What does participation mean to you? (Probe: What does it mean to
   fully participate in life?)
2. What areas of everyday life are most important to you to participate in?
   Is there anything in your life that, if it were taken away, would feel like a
   major participation loss?
3. What issues or barriers most affect your participation?
4. What are your biggest supports to participation?
5. What strategies (individual, social, societal, policy) are most needed to
   promote and support full participation?

RESULTS

Participation is a multifaceted, transactive process that involves interaction with the physical, social, cultural, attitudinal, and political environments. Members of the disability community expressed a desire to shape and contribute to those environments through meaningful participation.

Several themes related to core participation values emerged across the focus groups:

1. Active and meaningful engagement/being a part of
   - Participating in and being a part of an activity, context, social scene, or social group was based on feelings of safety and security.
   - Participants distinguished engagement from functionally independent performance.
   - There is a dynamic interaction between a person's willingness to take risks and the opportunities that society and the immediate social context afford people with disabilities.
   - "As a person with a disability or any other person, you don't have to follow that same path to somebody else's definition of fully participating, but you should have the opportunity or the option" (Hammel et al., p. 1450).
2. Choice and control
   - Risk-taking was closely tied to concepts of choice and control over the decision of how and when to participate.
   - Participants distinguished managing and controlling participation from independent activity performance.
   - To fully participate means to be able to self-advocate.
   - Full participation encompasses collective power, control, and voice in society for disabled people as a social group—moving beyond simply meeting individual needs.
   - "Nothing about us without us" (Hammel et al., p. 1451)
3. Access and opportunity/enfranchisement
   - Power is intimately related to societal access and opportunity at the person or group level.
   - Access and opportunities were closely related to participants' rights to social inclusion; contributions of disabled people were oftentimes overlooked or minimized.
   - People with disabilities do not want to be treated as inspirational, special, or seen as a charity case; this social construct of disability limits opportunities for engagement.

- People with disabilities should have the right to resources that support full participation because education and information are essential for decision-making (i.e., quality healthcare, assistive technology, and income assistance are prerequisites to participation).
- Participation is influenced by access to reasonable accommodations, including reliable, accessible, and affordable transportation.
- Able-bodied people should not make assumptions about the needs of those with disabilities; disabled people want to be recognized as experts of their needs and would like to be consulted in the design of accommodations.
- People in society treat those with disabilities as if their impairments in one area of function invalidate their abilities or access to opportunity in other areas (spread factor).
- "When they see me in a wheelchair, they talk to me like I'm deaf. I say I'm not deaf, my speech is impaired and I can't walk that fast but I'm not deaf. I'm in a wheelchair" (Hammel et al., p. 1452).

4. Personal and societal responsibilities
   - Participation is a responsibility to oneself and to one's family, community, and society in general.
   - Participation was defined by what those with disabilities can do to contribute to their communities and to others, not by what they can get from other people.
   - There is a reciprocal need for people with disabilities and societal responsibility in supporting their participation choice through equitable opportunities and resources.
   - "First you got to have positive thinking. And second you've got to say, you know, believe that there is nothing that you can't do. And then the third thing is just to get up and start doing it" (Hammel et al., p. 1452).

5. Having an impact and supporting others
   - Moving beyond personal productivity, social impact, and commitment were described as a need and a strong belief that permeated many participants' basic values and heavily influenced their behavior.
   - "The thing I found and I think it is a nice secret to learn, the way you do it is invest yourself in other people" (Hammel et al., p. 1453).

6. Social connection, societal inclusion, and membership
   - The social component of participation spanned from the highly personal and intimate to the very public and socially conscious; participation could mean friendships, companionships, and trusting relationships with others.
   - There is a lack of information about alternative forms of sexual expression when living with a disability, which limits opportunities for satisfying intimate relationships and sexual engagement.

- Religious or spiritual faith is another deeply personal form of connection.
- Disabled people do not want to be limited in only developing communities with other disabled people: "segregation is not a good idea."
- Being a member of a disability community and networking with others "like them" is important in creating a sense of shared understanding, strength, and community that creates opportunities for participation.
- Relationships with other people in the community . . . [also] relationships in the disability community, and role models with disabilities . . . are really important" (Hammel et al., p. 1453).

7. Respect and dignity (meta theme which emerged throughout the study and was identified as a critical feature of participation across all themes)
   - People with disabilities want to be treated with respect and dignity, including being seen as a person of value in communities and in the society at large.
   - Preference is to have respect from others, rather than acceptance of a disability.
   - Participants placed responsibility on society to respect and accommodate their differences, moving away from the individual remediation to environmental negotiation of participation.
   - Disability identity turned into a form of strength, pride, and culture.
   - "Instead of making us feel like we're lower class citizen, we should have our own new way to participate so that people CAN LEARN FROM US (emphasis added by speaker)" (Hammel et al., p. 1454).

Criticisms and Limitations: The study does not reflect the diversity of participation values of people in different cultural, political, and global contexts. The participants may represent a particularly informed and socially integrated sample of people with disabilities since they were recruited from state-of-the-art rehabilitation hospitals and centers for independent living in the United States.

Other Relevant Studies and Information:

- Eight major environmental factors influence participation: built, natural, transportation, assistive technology, information and technology access, social support and societal attitudes, systems and policies, and economics. Yet, the rehabilitation frame of reference only focuses on the immediate physical environment, which may be insufficient because community- and society-level factors are dynamic and have cumulative effects on participation (Angell et al., 2020).

- Occupational therapy practitioners can partner with local disability advocacy communities to support a sense of identity and self-confidence when discharge from hospital or institution to the community occurs (Angell et al., 2020).
- Considering human rights and human development perspectives, participation is one of the most important outcomes for children with disabilities and their families (Schlebusch et al., 2020).

Summary and Implications: Among persons with disabilities, participation not only includes active engagement in life situations at the societal level but also the personal meaning and satisfaction resulting from that engagement. The findings challenge researchers to critically examine conventional means of measuring participation via performance of a standard set of roles and activities that do not make sense for all people, who have different abilities, needs, and resources. The medical-rehabilitation field needs subjective and value-based participation assessment tools, reflecting a non-hierarchical conceptualization of participation created with the voice of the disability communities. Researchers should examine the complexity of participation in diverse social relationships, groups, communities, and cultures; the intricate role the environment plays in facilitating, obstructing, or transforming participation; and the allocation of resources so that people with disabilities can pursue "full" participation as they define it.

CLINICAL CASE: STILL DEPENDENT AND NEEDING TOTAL ASSIST AFTER 2 MONTHS IN REHABILITATION

Case History

Walid (he/him), a young man studying political science, is in an acute in-patient rehabilitation setting for a complete cervical level spinal cord injury after a car accident. The occupational therapist must demonstrate that he is making progress during inpatient rehabilitation as justification for hospitalization for the insurance company. The therapist is completing Section GG of the CARE tool, as required by the insurance company. Upon admission, the therapist scores Walid as "1" (Dependent) with all areas of self-care (eating, oral hygiene, toilet hygiene, shower, upper body dressing, lower body dressing, and putting on/taking off footwear). Two months later, the therapist is documenting a discharge level for all self-care categories and scores the patient as "1" (Dependent). The insurance company wants to deny payment because the patient did not make progress in therapy. What should the occupational therapist do?

Suggested Answer

The occupational therapist should document more than basic objective data that correlate to physical assistance that is required by a helper, as indicated in Section GG, or any other standardized assessment familiar to practitioners in this setting, such as the Functional Independence Measure or the Barthel Index. Utilizing the Occupational Therapy Practice Framework, the occupational therapist must intervene in areas that support occupations, including education, training, advocacy, and self-advocacy. The therapist should indicate the interdependence that Walid has experienced by learning how to self-advocate during self-care tasks and participating in meaningful activity by directing his own care and successfully communicating his needs to his caregivers to accomplish the necessary tasks for the day. Documentation should include the understanding and integration of patient learning and information that is life-saving, like knowing when to call for help if symptoms of autonomic dysreflexia occur or to facilitate pressure relief to avoid pressure injuries. Documentation should include peer support and mentorship from other people with disabilities, who have completed rehabilitation programs for cervical spinal cord injuries and have psychologically adjusted to their new lives and new bodies. It is critical to document not only physical assistance levels for basic self-care but also Walid's lived experience, including (but not limited to) safety and emergency maintenance, social and emotional health promotion and maintenance, symptom and condition management, communication with the healthcare system, medication and nutrition management, personal care device management, as well as rest and sleep, which are occupation-based areas not always captured in standardized assessments.

References

Angell, A. M., Goodman, L., Walker, H. R., McDonald, K. E., Kraus, L. E., Elms, E. H. J., Frieden, L., Sheth, Alisa J., & Hammel, J. (2020). "Starting to live a life": Understanding full participation for people with disabilities after institutionalization. *American Journal of Occupational Therapy, 74*, 7404205030p1–7404205030p11. https://doi.org/10.5014/ajot.2020.038489

Hammel, J., Magasi, S., Heinemann, H., Whiteneck, G., Bogner, J., & Rodriguez, E. (2008). What does participation mean? An insider perspective from people with disabilities. *Disability and Rehabilitation, 30*(19), 1445–1460. https://doi.org/10.1080/09638280701625534

Schlebusch, L., Huus, K., Samuels, A., Granlund, M., & Dada, S. (2020). Participation of young people with disabilities and/or chronic conditions in low- and middle-income countries: A scoping review. *Developmental Medicine & Child Neurology, 62,* 1259–1265. https://doi.org/10.1111/dmcn.14609

46

Cognitive Orientation to Daily Occupational Performance's (CO-OP's) Effectiveness in the Subacute Stroke Population

KELSEY PETERSON

CO-OP was associated with a large treatment effect on follow-up performances of self-selected activities and demonstrated transfer to untrained activities.

McEwen, S., Polatajko, H., Baum, C., Rios, J., Cirone, D., Doherty, M., & Wolf, T. (2015). Combined cognitive-strategy and task-specific training improve transfer to untrained activities in subacute stroke: An exploratory randomized controlled trial. *Neurorehabilitation and Neural Repair, 29*(6), 526–536.

Original Paper: https://doi.org/10.1177/1545968314558602

Research Question: How effective is the CO-OP approach in improving activity and participation for people less than 3 months post-stroke when compared to usual outpatient occupational therapy (OT) intervention?

Funding: The Canadian Institutes of Health Research Open Operating Grant, St. John's Rehab Foundation, and the National Center for Medical Rehabilitation Research in the National Institute of Child Health and Human Development of the National Institutes of Health

Year Study Began: 2011

Year Study Published: 2015

Study Location: Toronto, ON, Canada; St. Louis, MO, USA

Who Was Studied: People who were less than 3 months post–ischemic stroke. Participants in the CO-OP cohort were

- 57.5 years old (mean)
- 40.1 days post-stroke (mean)
- 31.6% female
- 47.4% White, 52.6% African American

Who Was Excluded: People who suffered a hemorrhagic stroke, had other neurological diagnoses or major psychiatric illness, suffered moderate to severe aphasia, or were determined to have a cognitive impairment (Montreal Cognitive Assessment ≤21).

How Many Patients: 26

Study Overview: Participants were randomly allocated to two groups: usual outpatient OT treatment or outpatient CO-OP (Figure 46.1).

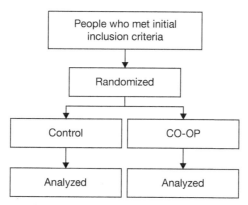

Figure 46.1 Participant design.

Study Intervention: Participants in the intervention group were treated by one CO-OP-trained occupational therapist (OT). Treatment sessions were 45 minutes and took place approximately twice per week. Participants were asked to select three goals from their initial Canadian Occupational Performance Measure (COPM) interview as the focus of subsequent intervention sessions. The OTs focused on the participants' implementation of the global cognitive strategy, goal–plan–do–check, to promote skill acquisition. An intervention fidelity checklist was utilized to score the fidelity of videotaped treatment sessions 3, 6, and 10.

The control group's OT sessions focused on functional, component-based, and task-based training. Treatment sessions lasted 45–60 minutes and were completed approximately twice per week. Session content was determined by the OTs' clinical reasoning. Results of the participants' COPM were provided, with no further direction given to the therapist.

Both the control and intervention groups received supplemental outpatient therapy as deemed necessary for their care (e.g., speech-language pathology, physical therapy, or nursing).

Follow-Up: Participants were tested at the first encounter, after 10 treatment sessions or discharge from OT ("post-intervention"), and 3 months after the completion of 10 sessions or discharge from OT ("3-month follow-up").

Endpoints: Primary outcome: Change in performance on Performance Quality Rating Scale (PQRS). Secondary outcomes: Perceived performance quality and satisfaction by the COPM; self-efficacy measured by the Self-Efficacy Gauge; participation, measured via the Community Participation Index and the Stroke Impact Scale participation domain.

RESULTS

- At post-intervention, CO-OP compared to usual care had a medium effect size for PQRS trained activities.
- At post-intervention, CO-OP compared to usual care had a large effect for PQRS untrained activities.
- At post-intervention, CO-OP compared to usual care had no effect on COPM change scores.
- At 3-month follow-up, CO-OP compared to usual care had large effect sizes for PQRS trained and untrained activities.
- At 3-month follow-up, CO-OP compared to usual care had medium effect sizes for change in participation via the Community Participation Index and self-efficacy.

Table 46.1. IMPACT OF CO-OP POST-INTERVENTION AND AT
3-MONTH FOLLOW-UP

Measure	Effect Size d[a] at Post-Intervention	Effect Size d at 3-Month Follow-Up
PQRS trained	0.5	1.6
PQRS untrained	1.2	1.1
COPM-performance trained	−0.1[b]	0.4
COPM-performance untrained	−0.1[b]	0.2
Control over participation[c]	N/A[d]	0.7
Self-Efficacy Gauge	0.4	0.7

N/A = not available.
[a]Effect size of 0.2 represents a small effect, 0.5 medium effect, and 0.8 large effect.
[b]No effect.
[c]Taken from results of the Community Participation Index.
[d]Unable to calculate as the measure is intended for people who have been in the community for a few weeks and thus was not administered at the first encounter with the participant.

Criticisms and Limitations: The sample size was small, which limited the ability to stratify groups on potential key confounders. The control arm was largely unstandardized, which may have led to differences among OT treatment sessions. The follow-up period was short, so it is not possible to ascertain the stability of the treatment effects beyond 3 months after discharge.

Other Relevant Studies and Information:

- CO-OP has also been demonstrated to improve self-perceived performance and performance satisfaction in the chronic stroke population (McEwen et al., 2009, 2010).
- Other studies have indicated that using the CO-OP approach is effective at improving transfer of skills in people of varying ages and diagnoses (Borujeni et al., 2019; Houldin et al., 2018).

Summary and Implications: For stroke survivors less than 3 months post–ischemic stroke, the CO-OP approach, compared to usual and customary outpatient OT, appears to improve participation in meaningful activities as well as transference of learned skills to untrained activities for at least 3 months following discharge from CO-OP. These results indicate that a larger trial analyzing the effects of the CO-OP approach on the post-stroke population is warranted.

CLINICAL CASE: CO-OP APPROACH WITH A PATIENT WITH RIGHT-SIDED WEAKNESS

Case History

Jae (he/him), a 54-year-old man with a history of hypertension and diabetes, presented to an acute care hospital after suffering an ischemic stroke at work. At the time of discharge, he required minimal assistance for his activities of daily living due to right-sided weakness. As such, it was recommended that he follow up in an outpatient OT clinic post-discharge.

Jae arrives at the OT outpatient clinic 30 days after his initial stroke. He is still having difficulty cleaning his home, making his bed, and cooking due to continued right-sided weakness. He tells the OT that he has been researching OT options for stroke survivors and found information about the CO-OP approach. He asks the OT if it would be a beneficial treatment approach during his time in outpatient therapy.

Suggested Answer

As Jae falls within the inclusion criteria for this study, he is likely to benefit from the CO-OP approach of utilizing the global cognitive strategy, goal–plan–do–check, to promote skill acquisition and improve his occupational performance. The CO-OP-trained OT should develop a plan of care emphasizing generalization of varying skills that would transfer to Jae's self-identified goals (i.e., cleaning the house, making his bed, cooking). Treatment sessions may focus on performance analysis and self-discovery of performance strategies through the plan and check phases of the CO-OP framework. This would allow the patient to work toward analyzing his own performance deficits and identifying his own strategies to improve his occupational performance across a variety of different tasks.

References

Borujeni, M. S., Hosseini, S. A., Akbarfahimi, N., & Ebrahimi, E. (2019). Cognitive orientation to daily occupational performance approach in adults with neurological conditions: A scoping review. *Medical Journal of the Islamic Republic of Iran, 33.* https://doi.org/10.34171/mjiri.33.99

Houldin, A., McEwen, S. E., Howell, M. W., & Polatajko, H. J. (2018). The cognitive orientation to daily occupational performance approach and transfer: A scoping review. *OTJR: Occupation, Participation, Health, 38*(3), 157–172. https://doi.org/10.1177/1539449217736059

McEwen, S. E., Polatajko, H. J., Huijbregts, M. P., & Ryan, J. D. (2009). Exploring a cognitive-based treatment approach to improve motor-based skill performance in chronic stroke: results of three single case experiments. *Brain Injury, 23*(13–14), 1041–1053. https://doi.org/10.3109/02699050903421107

McEwen, S. E., Polatajko, H. J., Huijbregts, M. P., & Ryan, J. D. (2010). Inter-task transfer of meaningful, functional skills following a cognitive-based treatment: Results of three multiple baseline design experiments in adults with chronic stroke. *Neuropsychological Rehabilitation, 20*(4), 541–561. https://doi.org/10.1080/09602011003638194

47

Development of a Client-Centered Occupational Performance Measure

PAMELA ROBERTS

COPM

The Canadian Occupational Performance Measure is an outcome measure for use by occupational therapists to assess client outcome in the areas of self-care, productivity and leisure.

LAW, M., BAPTISTE, S., McCOLL, M., OPZOOMER, A., POLATAJKO, H., & POLLOCK, N. (1990). The Canadian Occupational Performance Measure: An outcome measure for occupational therapy. *Canadian Journal of Occupational Therapy*, 57(2), 82–87.

Original Paper: https://doi.org/10.1177/000841749005700207

Research Question: What measure can evaluate and capture the important contributions of occupational therapy as described by the *Guidelines for the Client-Centered Practice of Occupational Therapy* (Department of National Health and Welfare [DNHW] & Canadian Association of Occupational Therapists [CAOT], 1983)?

Funding: The National Health Research and Development Programme of Health and Welfare Canada and the Canadian Occupational Therapy Foundation.

Year Study Began: 1988

Year Study Published: 1990

Study Location: Ontario, Canada

Who Was Studied: Clients across clinical practice areas in six communities across Ontario, Canada. Feedback from therapists who administered the instrument was also included.

Who Was Excluded: Not applicable. Study initially limited to six communities across Ontario, Canada, and was a convenience sample of clients across clinical practice areas. Not applicable

How Many Patients: 20

Study Overview: See Figure 47.1.

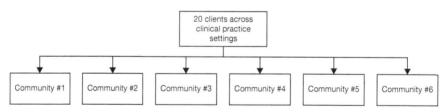

Figure 47.1. Overview of the study design.

Study Intervention: The Canadian Occupational Performance Measure (COPM) is a client-centered, criterion measure that reflects the philosophy of the model of occupational performance, by incorporating the roles and role expectations within the client's environment. The COPM framework is used to identify a client's perception of all areas of occupational performance including self-care, productivity, and leisure. Using a semi-structured interview, the information reflects the client's perception of their current level of occupational performance, their satisfaction with their performance, and the importance of the skill or activity. The COPM is designed to assist the occupational therapist (OT) in establishing occupational performance goals based on client perceptions of need and measures the change in defined problem areas. In this study, OTs administered the instrument across all practice settings in six communities.

Follow-Up: After completion of the pilot test and based on therapists' feedback, revisions were made to the COPM.

Endpoints: Development of an outcome measure that assists in structuring and focusing the OT assessment and intervention process.

RESULTS

- This study reports on the development of an outcome measure for use in occupational therapy.
- The COPM is an individualized measure of a client's self-perception of problems encountered in occupational performance using a semi-structured interview format and a structured scoring method.
- The COPM was designed to be used with the *Guidelines for a Client-Centered Practice of Occupational Therapy* (DNHW & CAOT, 1983)
- The COPM is intended to reflect the goals of individual clients and considers their roles and the environment. It asks the client to identify issues, rate their problems in terms of importance, rate their ability to perform the activity, and rate their current satisfaction level with their ability to perform the identified activities.
- The COPM is administered in a five-step process using a semi-structured interview. The steps are as follows: 1) problem identification in occupational performance areas of self-care, productivity, and leisure; 2) rating importance, performance, and satisfaction for each activity; 3) scoring to establish baseline scores that can be used for comparisons across time; 4) reassessment following the intervention process to evaluate change over time; and 5) follow-up to plan for intervention continuation or discharge.
- The COPM is a standardized outcome measure of occupational performance (participation in daily life context) and satisfaction with ability to perform life roles.
- The COPM provides the opportunity for the client to be a partner in their rehabilitation, provides a useful framework for initial assessment and reassessment of occupational performance, and bridges the client's priorities and the therapist's ideas for occupational therapy intervention.

Criticisms and Limitations: The initial pilot was completed in Ontario, Canada, in only six communities with 20 clients. In addition, the initial pilot did not include validity testing. Other limitations included identification of the timing of administration (e.g., whether to establish a relationship with the client before administering the measure), use of the COPM with caregivers including assessment of their ability to judge the importance of the activities to the client, and lack of direct observation of performance.

Other Relevant Studies and Information:

- Reliability testing revealed excellent test–retest reliability for performance and satisfaction and utility for use in community-based rehabilitation (Cup et al., 2003; Jenkinson et al., 2007).
- Validity was determined by comparing the COPM to other instruments and in a variety of populations (Cup et al., 2003; Harper et al., 2006; McColl et al., 2006; Chen et al., 2002; Thyer et al., 2018).
- A systematic review assessing the impact of the COPM in occupational therapy revealed that the greatest impact was in clinical practice (Parker & Sykes, 2006).
- Overall, multiple studies have shown that the COPM has efficient test–retest reliability, is appropriate for clinicians in assessing perceived outcome performance, and provides therapists with directions for interventions including goal development and intervention planning (Cup et al., 2003; Jenkinson et al., 2007; Harper et al., 2006; McColl et al., 2006; Chen et al., 2002; Thyer et al., 2018; Parker & Sykes, 2006; Doig et al., 2010).

Summary and Implications: The COPM is an outcome measure that uses a semi-structured interview that can be used in a wide variety of clinical settings. The COPM assists OTs to set goals and detect change with clients in perceived occupational performance over time.

CLINICAL CASE: GRACE AND USE OF ART IN THE ACUTE HOSPITAL

Case History

Grace (she/her), a 76-year-old retired artist, was referred to OT in an acute care hospital following a cerebrovascular accident (CVA). Prior to admission, Grace lived independently and taught art classes in the community. When the OT started the evaluation, Grace was withdrawn and not interested in getting out of bed or participating in basic self-care activities. The OT integrated the COPM into her assessment for identification of occupational performance problems in the areas of self-care, productivity, and leisure. During the COPM interview, the OT discovered that Grace was depressed after the stroke and fearful about losing the ability to take care of herself and teach art classes due to her right hand coordination deficits and loss of balance while standing. How might the OT use the COPM findings to develop a plan of care that addresses Grace's goals and priorities?

Suggested Answer

The COPM is a semi-structured interview between the client and the occupational therapist. Prior to integration of the COPM into the OT evaluation, Grace was withdrawn and disengaged. Through the COPM's occupation-based approach, Grace became motivated to participate in OT treatment focusing on self-care, functional mobility, and the use of art to address identified deficits in balance and fine motor coordination after the stroke. The occupational therapist positioned a large piece of paper on the wall that allowed Grace to engage in painting, her favorite occupation, while remediating deficits in balance and coordination. The use of the COPM enabled the occupational therapist to engage Grace and address the resultant deficits caused by the stroke in ways that were important and meaningful to the client.

References

Chen, Y. H., Rodger, S., & Polatajko, H. J. (2002). Experiences with the COPM and client-centered practice in adult neurorehabilitation in Taiwan. *Occupational Therapy International, 9*(3), 167–184. https://doi.org/10.1002/oti.163

Cup, E. H. C., Scholte, W. J. M., op Reimer, M. C. E., Thijssen, M. C. E., & van Kuyk-Minis, M. A. H. (2003). Reliability and validity of the Canadian Occupational Performance Measure in stroke patients. *Clinical Rehabilitation, 17*(4), 402–409. https://doi.org/10.1191/0269215503cr635oa

Department of National Health and Welfare & Canadian Association of Occupational Therapists. (1983). *Guidelines for the client-centered practice of occupational therapy* (H39-33/1983E).

Doig, E., Fleming, J., Lulpers, P., & Cornwell, P. L. (2010). Clinical utility of the combined use of the Canadian Occupational Performance Measure and Goal Attainment Scaling. *American Journal of Occupational Therapy, 64,* 904–914. https://doi.org/10.5014/ajot.2010.08156

Harper, K., Stalker, C. A., & Templeton, G. (2006). The use and validity of the Canadian Occupational Performance Measure in a posttraumatic stress program. *OTJR: Occupation, Participation & Health, 26*(2), 45–55.

Jenkinson, N., Ownsworth, T., & Shum, D. (2007). Utility of the Canadian Occupational Performance Measure in community-based brain injury rehabilitation. *Brain Injury, 21*(12), 1283–1294. https://doi.org/10.1080/02699050701739531

McColl, M. A., Carswell, A., Law, M., Pollock, N., Baptiste, S., & Polatajko, H. (2006). *Research on the Canadian Occupational Performance Measure: An annotated resource.* CAOT Publications ACE.

Parker, D. M., & Sykes, C. H. (2006). A systematic review of the Canadian Occupational Performance Measure: A clinical practice perspective. *British Journal of Occupational Therapy, 69*(4), 150–158.

Thyer, L., Brown, T., & Roe, D. (2018). The validity of the Canadian Occupational Performance Measure (COPM) when used in a sub-acute rehabilitation setting with older adults. *Occupational Therapy Health Care, 32*(2), 137–153. https://doi.org/10.1080/07380577.2018.1446233

48

Exploring the Association Between Therapy Time and Functional Recovery Through Mobility and Self Care Clinical Outcomes

KATIE JORDAN

In this study, rate of recovery and LOS [length of stay] in skilled nursing and inpatient rehabilitation facilities were associated with mobility and self-care outcomes at discharge following hip fracture surgery, particularly for medium-gain [based on scored improvements in self-care and mobility from admission to discharge] patients. Therapy time per day explained only 1% of the variance in discharge outcome. Discharging medium-gain patients before 21 days LOS may transfer burden of care to family and caregivers, home health, and outpatient services.

COGAN, A., WEAVER, J., MCHARG, M., LELAND, N. E., DAVIDSON, L., & MALLINSON, T. (2020). Association of Length of Stay, Recovery Rate, and Therapy Time per Day With Functional Outcomes After Hip Fracture Surgery. *JAMA Network Open, 3*(1), Article e1919672.

Original Paper: https://doi.org/10.1001/jamanetworkopen.2019.19672

Research Question: What is the association between therapy minutes per hospitalized day and functional recovery as captured by mobility and self-care clinical outcomes for patients engaged in rehabilitation in a post–acute care (PAC) setting (inpatient rehabilitation facility [IRF] or skilled nursing facility [SNF]) following surgery for a hip fracture?

Funding: Department of Education, National Institute on Disability, and Rehabilitation Research and Training Center on Measuring Rehabilitation Outcomes and Effectiveness

Year Study Began: 2005

Year Study Published: 2020

Study Location: Eastern and Midwestern United States

Who Was Studied: Participants who met inclusion criteria following surgery for a hip fracture coupled with PAC for rehabilitation services in multisite PAC settings: four IRFs and seven SNFs.

Who Was Excluded: Participants met the inclusion criteria if they were 1) admitted to an included PAC facility following surgery for a hip fracture, 2) 65 years old (or older), 3) eligible for and received therapy services, 4) insured by Medicare part B (fee-for-service), and 5) had complete records of their admission and discharge.

How Many Patients: 150

Study Overview: The findings of this study are based on a retrospective secondary analysis of multicenter prospective observational cohort data collected from 2005 to 2010 and analyzed from 2018 to 2019. Complete demographics, health condition and comorbidity information, and functional assessment measures were collected from admission and discharge medical records of study participants. Statistical analysis using Strata software (version 15.1) was completed to determine the relationships between patient characteristics, LOS (days hospitalized), therapy minutes, self-care, and mobility functional outcome scores (Figure 48.1).

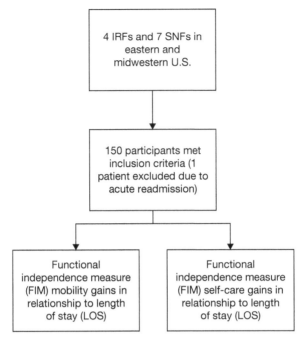

Figure 48.1. Overview of the study design.

Study Intervention: Not applicable

Follow-Up: Not applicable

Endpoints: Self-care and mobility gains as measured by the Functional Independence Measure (FIM).

RESULTS

- Patients were categorized into nine recovery groups to analyze the association between therapy minutes per LOS day (TMLD) and rate of functional gains.
  - Cut points for TMLD were established based on IRF and SNF rules.
  - Cut points for functional gains were established based on predicted levels of independence using the FIM as low (in need of assistance),

medium (some assistance required), or high (independence or modified independence) (Table 48.1).

- Functional mobility status was significantly different for each group on discharge but did not differ significantly on admission. Within each mobility gain group (low, medium, and high), TMLD was weakly associated with discharge status, while LOS was the most significant factor.
- Self-care status at discharge was significantly different for each group but did not differ significantly on admission or by facility (SNF vs. IRF). Gain group and LOS were most strongly associated with self-care measure score on discharge, but the difference between TMLD groups was statistically significant.
- Gains in functional outcomes were more strongly associated with LOS than with TMLD, which indicates that decisions around prioritization of patients, plan of care, dose, and intensity can and should be adjusted based on clinical judgment. Evidence-informed guidance can support value-based rehabilitation models. Some specific examples are listed below.
  - *Mobility considerations*
    - Participants in a low-gain trajectory never reached the level of mobility in the high-gain groups regardless of LOS or TMLD.
    - Participants in a high-gain trajectory for mobility with low TMLD had an extended LOS (average of 7 additional days) compared to those with high TMLD.
  - *Self-care considerations*
    - Participants in the medium- and high-gain trajectories performed better in self-care than the low-gain group when controlling for TMLD, three or more comorbidities, and LOS.
    - Most participants were grouped together for both mobility and self-care gains. If they were low for mobility, they were more likely low for self-care.
  - *LOS considerations*
    - Participants in a low-gain trajectory for both self-care and mobility with medium or high TMLD would likely achieve greater functional independence with less therapy if allowed a longer LOS.
    - Participants in the medium-gain trajectory for both self-care and mobility would likely achieve greater functional independence resulting in lower caregiver burden if LOS was extended beyond 21 days.

Table 48.1. RECOVERY GROUP DESIGNATIONS AS INTERSECTIONS OF TMLD AND FIM SCORES

| | | Gain in FIM Scores (Mobility and Self-Care) | | |
		Low	Medium	High
TMLD	Low	1 • Low TMLD • Low gain	2 • Low TMLD • Medium gain	3 • Low TMLD • High gain
	Medium	4 • Medium TMLD • Low gain	5 • Medium TMLD • Medium gain	6 • Medium TMLD • High gain
	High	7 • High TMLD • Low gain	8 • High TMLD • Medium gain	9 • High TMLD • High gain

Criticisms and Limitations: As this was a retrospective study and a secondary data analysis with a small sample size, there are limitations. The timing, quality, and content of the therapy provided beyond the number of minutes were not available. Functional status was assessed at two points in time (admission and discharge) and, therefore, could not be tracked over the course of the plan of care.

Other Relevant Studies and Information:

- Recovery from hip fracture repair in PAC settings, specifically SNF, IRF, and home health (HH), is difficult to compare given the variability in therapy intensity and dose, LOS, and outcome measure tools between types of settings (Mallinson et al., 2014).
- Patients are admitted to PAC settings (SNF, IRF, HH) based on characteristics such as rehabilitation potential, comorbidities, and level of home and community support, as well as medical severity. However, patients discharged home following lower extremity joint replacement surgery achieved greater functional gains after HH services when compared to patients who were discharged to IRF and SNF (while controlling for comorbidities, demographic characteristics, and social support), suggesting that the home environment may provide a better rehabilitation opportunity in a more natural context (Mallinson et al., 2011).
- Risk factors including readmission and care process transition issues must be considered and may be impacted by decisions of PAC settings including therapy dose, content, intensity, LOS, and modifiable patient

characteristics (functional status including self-care and mobility) (Gerrard et al., 2015; Kumar et al., 2018).

- In a study reviewing over 1.4 million Medicare cases, occupational therapy and physical therapy were found to be associated with greater increases in patient functioning and reductions in hospital readmissions. (AOTA & APTA, 2021)

Summary and Implications: Critical decisions regarding allocation of therapy resources in PAC settings are generally based on regulatory and reimbursement requirements. Using retrospective data, this study provides statistical evidence to demonstrate that rate of functional gain (mobility and self-care scores) and LOS were more strongly associated with functional outcomes at discharge than therapy minutes provided to patients receiving rehabilitation in a PAC setting (SNF or IRF) following hip fracture surgery. Importantly, this study provides strong evidence to support the consideration of patient characteristics, anticipated LOS, caregiver burden, and clinical reasoning in determining the most cost-effective and clinically optimal rehabilitation plan of care. This approach is invaluable as we move from fee-for-service to value-based care in all healthcare contexts.

CLINICAL CASE: HIP FRACTURE RECOVERY TRAJECTORY

Case History

Elaina (she/her), a 78-year-old female, is briefly admitted to an orthopedic acute care unit for recovery following a hip fracture surgery after a fall in her apartment. The occupational therapist evaluating the patient completes an occupational profile, considering her medical and therapy history prior to this admission. Elaina has eight comorbidities including bladder incontinence, mild cognitive impairment, and vision impairment; lives independently with one short flight of stairs to get into her apartment; has no community-level social or family support; and was previously independent in mobility and self-care. This patient is admitted to an SNF for rehabilitation.

Suggested Answer

This patient vignette is typical of cases reviewed in this study. With no caregiver support, it is critical that Elaina regain functional independence in both self-care and mobility. If she is assessed to be on a high-gain self-care and mobility trajectory at the SNF, the therapists could decrease therapy minutes and expect that she would be able to return home if LOS is 18–20 days. However, if Elaina is assessed to be on a medium-gain trajectory, therapists may need to increase therapy minutes and LOS may need to be extended to 21 days or more in order to return home. If the patient is on a low-gain trajectory, it is unlikely that she will be able to return home independently regardless of therapy minutes or LOS, and the team should recommend a higher level of long-term care.

References

American Occupational Therapy Association & American Physical Therapy Association. (2021). *Therapy outcomes in post–acute care settings: Study summary.* https://www.aota.org/-/media/Corporate/Files/Advocacy/Federal/tops/TOPS-Study-Summary.pdf

Gerrard, P., Goldstein, R., DiVita, M. A., Slocum, C., Ryan, C. M., Mix, J., Niewczyk, P., Kazis, L., Zafonte, R., & Schneider, J. C. (2015). Functional status and readmissions in unilateral hip fractures. *American Journal of Managed Care, 21*(4), e282–e287.

Kumar, A., Rahman, M., Trivedi, A. N., Resnik, L., Gozalo, P., & Mor, V. (2018). Comparing post-acute rehabilitation use, length of stay, and outcomes experienced by Medicare fee-for-service and Medicare Advantage beneficiaries with hip fracture in the United States: A secondary analysis of administrative data. *PLoS Medicine, 15*(6), Article e1002592. https://doi.org/10.1371/journal.pmed.1002592

Mallinson, T. R., Bateman, J., Tseng, H.-Y., Manheim, L., Almagor, O., Deutsch, A., & Heinemann, A. W. (2011). A comparison of discharge functional status after rehabilitation in skilled nursing, home health, and medical rehabilitation settings for patients after lower-extremity joint replacement surgery. *Archives of Physical Medicine and Rehabilitation, 92*(5), 712–720. https://doi.org/10.1016/j.apmr.2010.12.007

Mallinson, T., Deutsch, A., Bateman, J., Tseng, H.-Y., Manheim, L., Almagor, O., & Heinemann, A. W. (2014). Comparison of discharge functional status after rehabilitation in skilled nursing, home health, and medical rehabilitation settings for patients after hip fracture repair. *Archives of Physical Medicine and Rehabilitation, 95*(2), 209–217. https://doi.org/10.1016/j.apmr.2013.05.031

49

Early Occupational and Physical Therapy for Critically Ill Patients Requiring Mechanical Ventilation

PHUONG NGUYEN

A strategy for whole-body rehabilitation—consisting of interruption of sedation and physical and occupational therapy in the earliest days of critical illness—was safe and well tolerated, and resulted in better functional outcomes at hospital discharge, a shorter duration of delirium, and more ventilator-free days compared with standard care.

SCHWEICKERT, W. D., POHLMAN, M. C., POHLMAN, A. S., NIGOS, C., PAWLIK, A. J., ESBROOK, C. L., SPEARS, L., MILLER, M., FRANCZYK, M., DEPRIZIO, D., SCHMIDT, G. A., BOWMAN, A., BARR, R., MCCALLISTER, K. E., HALL, J. B., & KRESS. J. P. (2009). Early physical and occupational therapy in mechanically ventilated, critically ill patients: A randomised controlled trial. *Lancet, 373*(9678), 1874–1882.

Original Paper: https://doi.org/10.1016/S0140-6736(09)60658-9

Research Question: Does early occupational and physical therapy improve functional and health outcomes for critically ill, mechanically ventilated patients?

Funding: None

Year Study Began: 2005

Year Study Published: 2009

Study Location: Chicago, IL; Iowa City, IA

Who Was Studied: Adults admitted to the intensive care unit (ICU) who

- Had been on mechanical ventilation for less than 72 hours and expected to continue for at least 24 hours
- Met baseline functional independence (Barthel Index score ≥70 two weeks before admission)

Who Was Excluded: Adults with rapidly developing neuromuscular disease, cardiopulmonary arrest, irreversible disorders with 6-month mortality, raised intracranial pressure, or absent limbs or who were enrolled in another trial.

How Many Patients: 104

Study Overview: See Figure 49.1.

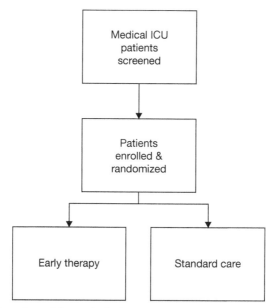

Figure 49.1. Overview of the study design.

Study Intervention: Patients in the intervention group received occupational and physical therapy as early as possible once they were identified to have met criteria and enrolled in the study. Therapy was coordinated to occur daily with sedation interruption. Unresponsive patients were provided passive range of motion for all limbs. Interactive patients would receive therapy that progressed based on tolerance: active assisted and active range of motion in supine, bed mobility (e.g., sitting upright), seated level activities (e.g., activities of daily living [ADLs], exercises), transfer training (e.g., bed to chair or commode), pre-gait exercises, and walking. Interventions continued until the patient reached baseline function or was discharged.

Patients in the control group received occupational and physical therapy per standard care and daily sedation interruption. Standard care therapy was ordered at the discretion of the medical team, where therapy was not routinely provided for patients on mechanical ventilation for less than 2 weeks.

Follow-Up: Patients were assessed at baseline, every 48 hours, and within 24 hours of discharge.

Endpoints:

Primary outcome: The number of patients returning to an independent functional status at time of discharge (i.e., able to perform six ADLs and walk without physical assistance).

Secondary outcomes: Duration of delirium and ventilator-free days within the first 28 days of the hospital stay.

RESULTS

- Overall, 29 of the 49 patients (59%) in the intervention group returned to independent functional status at hospital discharge compared to 19 of the 55 patients (35%) in the control group.
- The appreciable effect of the intervention on functional status was delayed by approximately 2 weeks, at which time functional status plateaued within the control group and continued to improve within the intervention group.
- The intervention group had a shorter duration of ICU-associated delirium (2.0 fewer days) and mechanical ventilation (2.7 fewer days) compared to the control group.

- There was no significant difference in ICU or hospital length of stay between the intervention and control groups.
- The intervention group received occupational and physical therapy for a median of 0.32 hours per day, with treatment initiated at 1.5 days post-intubation, compared to the control group at 0.0 hours per day and initiation at 7.4 days post-intubation.
- Serious adverse events were rare, with only one serious adverse event (oxygen desaturation <80%) and one inadvertent removal of a radial artery catheter in the intervention group occurring in 498 occupational and physical therapy sessions over 2 years.
- Patients in the intervention group had higher Barthel Index scores (75/100 vs. 55/100), higher number of independent ADLs (6 vs. 4), and greater walking distance (33.4 vs. 0 m) at hospital discharge compared to those in the control group.
- Patients in the intervention group trended toward better discharge rates to home than the control group (43% vs. 24%, $p = 0.06$), which may support the notion that early mobilization can reduce post–acute rehabilitation care cost (Table 49.1).

Table 49.1. SUMMARY OF STUDY'S KEY FINDINGS

Outcome	Intervention Group Early Therapy (n = 49)	Control Group Standard Care (n = 55)	p
Return to independent functional status at hospital discharge (n, %)	29 (59%)	19 (35%)	0.02
Barthel Index score at hospital discharge (out of 100)	75 (7.5–95)	55 (0–85)	0.05
ICU delirium (days)	2.0 (0.0–6.0)	4.0 (2.0–7.0)	0.03
Duration of mechanical ventilation (days)	3.4 (2.3–7.3)	6.1 (4.0–9.6)	0.02
Length of stay in ICU (days)	5.9 (4.5–13.2)	7.9 (6.1–12.9)	0.08
Discharge to home (n, %)	21 (43%)	13 (24%)	0.06

Criticisms and Limitations: This study was conducted with a specific group of critically ill patients requiring mechanical ventilation (i.e., previously independent; diagnoses not specified), so the results cannot be assumed to be applicable to all mechanically ventilated patients. In addition, the nature of the intervention required adjusting to individual patients' needs and medical statuses and, as such, did not control for timing and dose of interventions and prevented blinding from patients and other members of the healthcare team. Therefore, there was a potential for knowledge of group allocation and a risk of bias in the results.

Other Relevant Studies and Information:

- With judicious clinical assessment, early mobilization and therapy are safe and feasible with critically ill patients, including those diagnosed with COVID-19 (Doiron et al., 2018; Girard et al., 2017; Goodwin et al., 2021; Hodgson et al., 2014; Pun et al., 2018; Tipping et al., 2016; Weinreich et al., 2017).
- Early mobilization and intervention may contribute to improved patient outcomes, such as decreased hospital length of stay, decreased duration of mechanical ventilation and delirium, and improved functional status (Girard et al., 2017; Goodwin et al., 2021; Pun et al., 2018; Tipping et al., 2016; Weinreich et al., 2017).
- The quality of evidence for early mobilization or occupational and physical therapy is low to moderate, due to small sample sizes, lack of blinded interventions, and variability in interventions and assessments across studies (Doiron et al., 2018; Girard et al., 2017; Goodwin et al., 2021; Hodgson et al., 2014; Tipping et al., 2016; Weinreich et al., 2017).
- Though the quality of evidence is variable, clinical expert consensus recommends early mobility, intervention, and therapy for critically ill patients as it is generally safe and feasible and has the potential to improve outcomes (Girard et al., 2017; Goodwin et al., 2021; Hodgson et al., 2014).

Summary and Implications: For critically ill adult patients requiring mechanical ventilation, early exercise and mobilization provided by occupational and physical therapists was safe and improved outcomes. A greater percentage of patients receiving early intervention were discharged with an independent functional status and had shorter duration of delirium and mechanical ventilation. Though not all outcomes measured showed improvement or rose to the level of statistical significance, the intervention rarely (one occurrence) caused adverse events and showed positive outcomes for primary and secondary endpoints. Taken together, provided patients' preferences are aligned with the care team, this study supports the expert consensus that the benefits outweigh the risks for implementing an early rehabilitation strategy for critically ill, mechanically ventilated patients.

CLINICAL CASE: EARLY REHABILITATION DURING MECHANICAL VENTILATION

Case History

José (he/him), a 56-year-old male, presents to the emergency room with flu-like symptoms. Per his wife, José was in good health and performing his usual activities, including working as a mailman and helping with household chores, up until two days ago when he began to complain of chills, fever, body aches, and severe shortness of breath. His respiratory status rapidly declines, requiring José to be intubated and placed on mechanical ventilation. He is transferred to the ICU and diagnosed with acute respiratory distress syndrome. Based upon information available, would José benefit from early occupational therapy and physical therapy?

Suggested Answer

The deleterious effects of critical illness and immobility on patients, including physical, cognitive, and psychosocial deficits, are well documented. Schweickert et al., as well as many others, have demonstrated that early occupational therapy and physical therapy is a safe and feasible intervention to combat these issues. Though the quality of evidence is low to moderate (i.e., low sample size, lack of blinding, variable interventions) with inconsistent results, clinical expert consensus supports early intervention as this study and others demonstrate significant potential benefits countered by minimal risks to patients' health outcomes. In this case, the patient was functionally independent and in good health at baseline. Therefore, he appears to be a good candidate for early therapy and would benefit from occupational and physical therapy to progress his physical, cognitive, psychosocial, and functional gains. While considering and monitoring the patient's medical and respiratory status, occupational therapists could facilitate early mobilization and early engagement in light activities of daily living, social participation, and leisure, upright and out of bed, that would promote recovery of the whole body and mind.

References

Doiron, K., Hoffmann, T., & Beller, E. (2018). Early intervention (mobilization or active exercise) for critically ill adults in the intensive care unit. *Cochrane Database of Systematic Reviews*, (3), Article CD010754. https://doi.org/10.1002/14651858. CD010754.pub2

Girard, T.D., Alhazzani, W., Kress, J.P., Ouellette, D.R., Schmidt, G.A., Truwit, J.D., Burns, S. M., Epstein, S. K., Esteban, A., Fan, E., Ferrer, M., Fraser, G. L., Gong, M. N., Hough,

C. L., Mehta, S., Nanchal, R., Patel, S., Pawlik, A. J., Schweikert, W. D., . . . Morris, P.E. (2017). An official American Thoracic Society/American College of Chest Physicians clinical practice guideline: Liberation from mechanical ventilation in critically ill adults; rehabilitation protocols, ventilator liberation protocols, and cuff leak tests. *American Journal of Respiratory and Critical Care Medicine, 195*(1), 120–133.

Goodwin, V. A., Allan, L., Bethel, A., Cowley, A., Cross, J. L., Day, J., Drummond, A., Hall, A. J., Howard, M., Morley, N., Thompson Coon, J., & Lamb, S. E. (2021). Rehabilitation to enable recovery from COVID-19: A rapid systematic review. *Physiotherapy, 111*, 4–22. https://doi.org/10.1016/j.physio.2021.01.007

Hodgson, C.L., Stiller, K., Needham, D.M., Tipping, C.J., Harold, M., Baldwin, C.E., Bradley, S., Berney, S., Caruana, L. R., Elliott, D., Green, M., Haines, K., Higgins, A. M., Kaukonen, K.-M., Leditschke, I. A., Nickels, M. R., Paratz, J., Patman, S., Skinner, E. H., . . . Web, S. A. (2014). Expert consensus and recommendations on safety criteria for active mobilization of mechanically ventilated critically ill adults. *Critical Care, 18*, Article 658. https://doi.org/10.1186/s13054-014-0658-y

Pun, B.T., Balas, M.C., Barnes-Daly, M. A., Thompson, J.L., Aldrichk, J. M., Barr, J., Byrum, D., Carson, S. S., Devlin, J. W., Engel, H. J., Esbrook, C. L., Hargett, K. D., Harmon, L., Hielsberg, C., Jackson, J. C., Kelly, T. L., Kumar, V., Millner, L., Morse, A., . . . Ely, E. W. (2018). Caring for critically ill patients with the ABCDEF bundle: Results of the ICU Liberation Collaborative in over 15,000 adults. *Critical Care Medicine, 47*(1), 3–14. https://doi.org/10.1097/CCM.0000000000003482

Tipping, C.J., Harrold, M., Holland, A., Romero, L., Nisbet, T., & Hodgson, C.L. (2016). The effects of active mobilisation and rehabilitation in ICU on mortality and function: A systematic review. *Intensive Care Medicine, 43*, 171–183. https://doi.org/10.1007/s00134-016-4612-0

Weinreich, M., Herman, J., Dickason, S., & Mayo, H. (2017). Occupational therapy in the intensive care unit: A systematic review. *Occupational Therapy in Health Care, 31*(3), 205–213. https://doi.org/10.1080/07380577.2017.1340690

50

Occupational Therapy is the Cost-Effective Solution to Support High Quality Care and Reduce Readmissions in Hospitals

KATIE JORDAN

Using Medicare claims and cost report data, we examined the association between hospital spending for specific services and 30-day readmission rates for heart failure, pneumonia, and acute myocardial infarction. We found that occupational therapy is the only spending category where additional spending has a statistically significant association with lower readmission rates for all three medical conditions.
ROGERS, A. T., BAI, G., LAVIN, R. A., & ANDERSON, G. F. (2017). Higher hospital spending on occupational therapy is associated with lower readmission rates. *Medical Care Research and Review*, 74(6), 668–686.

Original Paper: https://journals.sagepub.com/doi/full/10.1177/107755871 6666981

Research Question: Which specific hospital spending categories, when provided with additional funding support, are correlated with improved (reduced) readmission rates for three clinical conditions included in the Medicare Hospital Readmission Reduction Program (HRRP)?

Funding: The authors received no financial support for this original research and/or for the authorship and publication of this article.

Year Study Began: 2009–2012

Year Study Published: 2017

Study Location: 7174 US hospitals

Who Was Studied: Patients who met criteria established by the Centers for Medicare and Medicaid Services (CMS) and HRRP: 1) Medicare fee-for-service enrollee; 2) age 65 or older; and 3) have been discharged from an acute care hospital (non-federal) with a primary diagnosis of heart failure (HF), acute myocardial infarction (AMI), or pneumonia (PN).

Who Was Excluded: Patients who 1) expired in the hospital and therefore could not be readmitted; 2) were admitted and discharged on the same day due to a clinically insignificant case of HF, AMI, or PN; 3) were transferred to another hospital since readmission is attributed to the discharging hospital; or 4) self-discharged against medical advice.

How Many Patients: 1,194,250

Study Overview: This study was a retrospective analysis of a large data set using publicly available hospital and CMS data, risk-adjusted by CMS to account for patient characteristics and comorbidities including indicators of frailty. The authors analyzed spending in 19 identified hospital spending categories (cost centers) to identify which were associated with readmission rates for patients with HF, PN, or AMI. Under the CMS HRRP, readmission of patients with these diagnoses results in a penalty to hospital reimbursement of up to 3%, or incentive payments are provided to hospitals that perform well on this quality indicator (Figure 50.1).

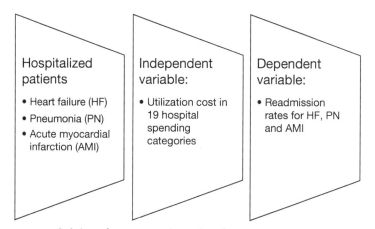

Figure 50.1. Probability of return to independent functional status.

Study Intervention: Nineteen identified hospital spending categories (cost centers), including occupational therapy and 18 other cost centers, both clinical (e.g., nursing, physical therapy) and operational (e.g., housekeeping, financial services).

Follow-Up: This study focused on national CMS data for 30-day readmission rates for patients discharged following HF, PN, and/or AMI.

Endpoints: Primary outcome for this study was 30-day readmission to the hospital for patients with a primary admitting diagnosis of HF, PN, or AMI. These diagnoses are included in the CMS HRRP and therefore subject to reimbursement penalty and incentive payments.

RESULTS

- Occupational therapy was the only spending category with a statistically significant negative association with hospital readmission for patients with HF, PN, and AMI. The authors speculate that this is likely due to occupational therapy focusing on self-care, cognitive and general function, and social determinants of health that typically affect readmission risk.
- Few patients in the study received occupational therapy services (HF, 26%; PN, 29%; AMI, 21%).
- Spending on cardiology and emergency room services following occupational therapy showed the second and third most statistically significant negative associations for hospital readmission, respectively.
- Average hospital spending for occupational therapy is relatively low ($12–$20) per patient (utilizing patient risk-adjusted costs for all admitted patients with HF, PN, or AMI, regardless of their receipt of occupational therapy services) (Table 50.1).

Table 50.1. SUMMARY OF KEY FINDINGS REGARDING OCCUPATIONAL THERAPY

Occupational Therapy	Percentage of Total Hospital Costs Assigned to OT	Percentage of Patients with Occupational Therapy Charges	Readmission Coefficient	Readmission SE	Readmission *p* Value
Heart failure (*n* = 2761)	0.3%	26.4%	−0.55	0.177	0.0018
Pneumonia (*n* = 2818)	0.4%	28.5%	−0.36	0.132	0.0068

Occupational Therapy	Percentage of Total Hospital Costs Assigned to OT	Percentage of Patients with Occupational Therapy Charges	Readmission Coefficient	Readmission SE	Readmission p Value
Acute myocardial infarction ($n = 1595$)	0.2%	21.1%	−0.68	0.295	0.0217

Criticisms and Limitations: Findings of this study relate to patients with HF, PN, and AMI specifically and may not, therefore, be generalizable to people with other primary diagnoses. The quality measures and data sets used, while validated by the National Quality Forum and CMS, have been criticized in the literature for lack of completeness. Analysis was based on observational data; therefore, conclusive statements about causality should be avoided.

Other Relevant Studies and Information:

- Evidence of the direction and strength of the relationship of cost to quality is largely inconsistent. Future studies should focus on the types of spending positively associated with quality and those affiliated with system waste (Hussey et al., 2013).
- Predictors and strategies to successfully mitigate readmission risk are multifactorial and rarely generalizable. "Post-hospital syndrome" describes a period of likely vulnerability where intervention may have a more positive impact (Dharmarajan et al., 2013; Dharmarajan & Krumholz, 2014).
- Occupational therapy practitioners in hospital-based practice are well positioned to positively affect clinical outcomes for vulnerable patients and hospital quality indicators including readmission (Roberts & Robinson, 2014).

Summary and Implications: Policy makers and health system leaders are under constant pressure to produce consistent, high-quality care that meets or exceeds patient expectations while remaining cost-effective. Existing literature tends to focus on aggregated cost or outcome, making it difficult to determine where the positive and negative impacts originate from, and therefore where de-cision makers should focus scarce and competing resources. Using large, national data sets, this study demonstrates that occupational therapy is the only hospital spending category that was consistently associated with lower rates of readmission for three HRRP diagnoses used to measure hospital readmission performance. With the cost of occupational therapy services relatively low among hospital cost centers and the majority of patients (72%–79%) not receiving occupational therapy services, this study provides clear guidance and evidence to support investment in hospital occupational therapy departments as a means to improve quality of care and reduce readmission rates, without significantly increasing hospital spending.

CLINICAL CASE: UTILIZATION OF OCCUPATIONAL THERAPY TO PROMOTE COST-EFFECTIVE HOSPITAL CARE

Case History

Livia (she/her), a 75-year-old woman, is admitted to an acute care hospital following a short emergency department (ED) stay with an admitting diagnosis of AMI. She lives in a one-story, single-family home with her spouse, who has mobility and functional impairments and for whom she is the primary caregiver. While she has a daughter who lives locally and is willing and available to assist, she was previously independent with all activities of daily living (ADLs), instrumental ADLs (IADLs) including driving, and functional mobility tasks. What services should Livia receive to most cost-effectively optimize her hospital stay and best prepare her for a safe and permanent discharge to her home and community?

Suggested Answer

In addition to occupational therapy, this study found that emergency and cardiology services were the second and third, respectively, most statistically significant services negatively associated with readmission. Once Livia is stabilized in the ED, her primary care team in acute care should include cardiology and occupational therapy. The occupational therapy intervention plan of care should address a wide range of factors that are likely to impact hospital readmission including, but not limited to, patient education, ADL (self-care and functional mobility) retraining, IADL retraining (community reintegration), home safety assessment, cognitive assessment and retraining as clinically indicated, activity tolerance/endurance following AMI, medication management, and comprehensive and integrated discharge planning with the care team and family.

References

Dharmarajan, K., Hsieh, A. F., Lin, Z., Bueno, H., Ross, J. S., Horwitz, L. I., Barreto-Filho, J. A., Kim, N., Bernheim, S. M., Suter, L. G., Drye, E. E., & Krumholz, H. M. (2013). Diagnoses and timing of 30-day readmissions after hospitalization for heart failure, acute myocardial infarction, or pneumonia. *Journal of the American Medical Association, 309*, 355–363.

Dharmarajan, K., & Krumholz, H. M. (2014). Strategies to reduce 30-day readmissions in older patients hospitalized with heart failure and acute myocardial infarction. *Current Geriatrics Reports, 3*, 306–315.

Hussey, P. S., Wertheimer, S., & Mehrotra, A. (2013). The association between health care quality and cost: A systematic review. *Annals of Internal Medicine, 158*, 27–34.

Roberts, P. S., & Robinson, M. R. (2014). Occupational therapy's role in preventing acute readmissions. *American Journal of Occupational Therapy, 68*, 254–259.

INDEX

For the benefit of digital users, indexed terms that span two pages (e.g., 52–53) may, on occasion, appear on only one of those pages.

Tables, figures, and boxes are indicated by *t*, *f*, and *b* following the page number